HARRY'S WAR

From Dunkirk to the Burma Railway

A Doctor's Diary

Harry Silman and Jacqueline Passman

Tambar

ISBN 978-1-910133-20-0

Tambar Arts Ltd: Reg. No. 03937329

www.tambar.co.uk

e-mail: contact@tambar.co.uk

Cover and book graphic design: Dylan Martin @ www.friedbanana.co.uk

Publication date: 15 August 2020 (75th Anniversary V-J Day)

For Miranda, Nick, Andrea,
Sara, Jo, Tim & Dan
in memory of
their much-loved Grandpa

Acknowledgements

This book was written at the prompting of my cousin Robert. I could not have accomplished it without his invaluable advice and encouragement as my editor. Special thanks are due to my daughter Miranda for her suggestions and accurate proof-reading. I am also grateful to my brother Alan for deciphering and explaining the obscure medical terms in the original diary, and my sister Marilyn for her constant support in everything I do.

Contents

Chapter One

Introduction

The core of this book are my father's diaries and letters, from his time with the army in France and his imprisonment in the Far East. These quotes are shown in *italics*.

There are several other sources throughout this book. I have given a note number for these other sources which are detailed in Appendix One.

Of particular significance are the observations by Harry in a documentary about him produced by Yorkshire Television in 2003 when he was 92 years old[1]; the research by Louise Reynolds, née Cordingly[2], and Paul Reynolds[3] who are the daughter and son-in-law of Padre Cordingly[4], Harry's friend and fellow POW; and the narrative by Jim Bradley[5], also a friend and fellow captive.

My father, Harry Silman, was born on 21 December 1910, the third of four children of Fanny and Reuben Silman in Leeds. Harry was educated at Leeds Grammar School and Leeds University where he studied medicine. After graduation he worked both as a general practitioner and at Leeds General Infirmary.

One of his first appointments was in a rural practice in Hawes in North Yorkshire. Here he conducted his rounds in a horse and cart, and was frequently paid in kind with foodstuffs from the farmers in his practice. This was in the 1930s before the creation of the National Health Service which introduced free medical care for all in 1948. As was common for doctors at this time, he also did his own dispensing. His two most effective prescriptions were placebos, one coloured blue and the other pink, with patients vowing that one worked much better than the other.

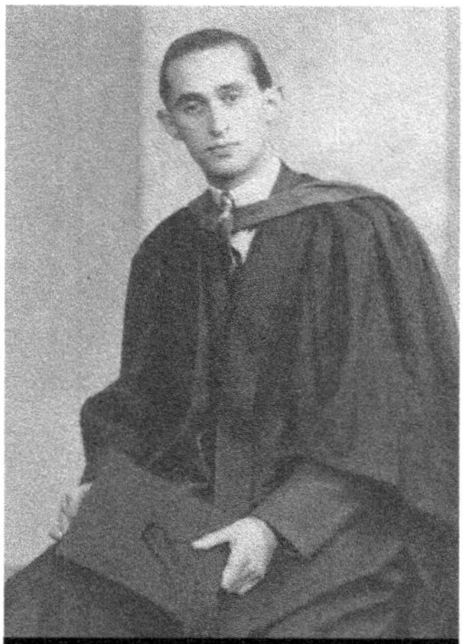

Harry Silman graduation

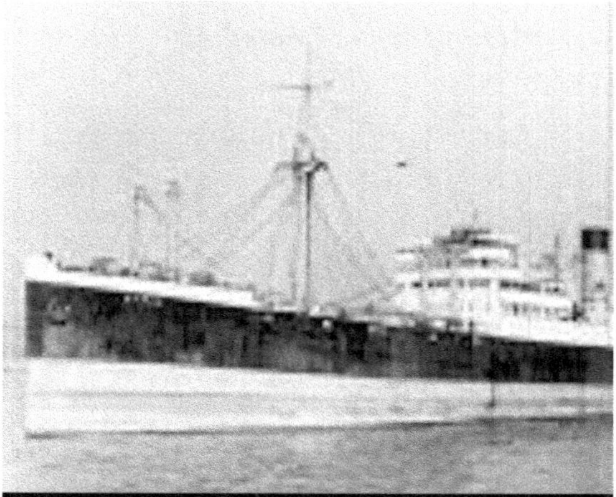

MS Glenbeg

A highlight of his pre-war medical years was his four months serving as the doctor on a cargo ship, MS *Glenbeg* in 1936. Merchant ships used to carry a few first-class passengers and, in addition to his medical duties, Harry was the co-ordinator for their on-board activities. This is Harry's description of one trip: *There are nine passengers viz: one married male – jovial and hearty – going out to plant rubber, by gad! and to shoot tigers, by Jove! Five married females going out to join their husbands in the far-flung corners of the empire and three single girls... bright young things who have to be kept well in hand.*

He described a small surgical operation on a sailor: *The patient, in spite of my telling him to have no food before the operation, took no notice and ate a hearty lunch. Consequently halfway through the operation he proceeded to vomit copiously. This combined with the smell of the pus, the make-shift hospital in a lumber room, the gallery of inquisitive Chinese sailors, and not forgetting the fact that the temperature was a hundred and plenty in the shade made the afternoon a memorable one. All my attempts at asepsis were quite nullified by well-meaning helpers who fingered all my sterile instruments. However, I am pleased to relate, the patient is still living and is doing well.*

After travelling through the Suez Canal, he saw a big Italian passenger ship anchored close by. *There were scenes of tremendous enthusiasm, cheering, clapping and waving of flags. I was told Mussolini's wife was on board, and all the Italian inhabitants of Suez had turned out to greet her.*

By a strange coincidence, Harry met the captain of the *Glenbeg*, six years later. Captain Newing was the pilot of the French ship *Felix Roussel* which took him into Singapore on 5th February 1942 and then left immediately, evacuating 1,100 Singapore civilians.

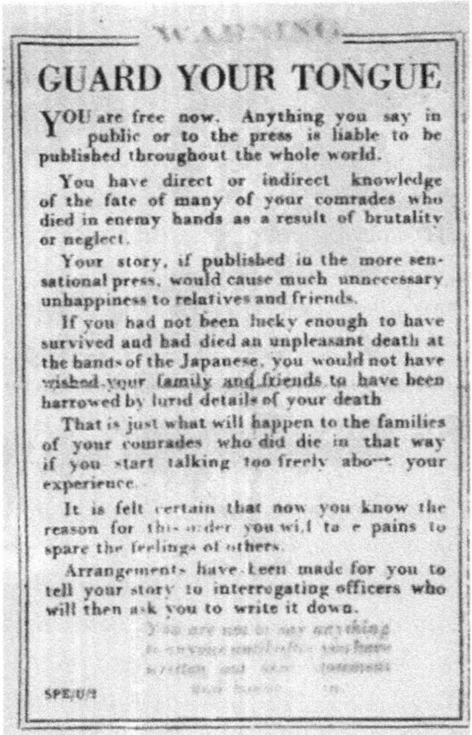

GUARD YOUR TONGUE

YOU are free now. Anything you say in public or to the press is liable to be published throughout the whole world.

You have direct or indirect knowledge of the fate of many of your comrades who died in enemy hands as a result of brutality or neglect.

Your story, if published in the more sensational press, would cause much unnecessary unhappiness to relatives and friends.

If you had not been lucky enough to have survived and had died an unpleasant death at the hands of the Japanese, you would not have wished your family and friends to have been harrowed by lurid details of your death.

That is just what will happen to the families of your comrades who did die in that way if you start talking too freely about your experience.

It is felt certain that now you know the reason for this order you will take pains to spare the feelings of others.

Arrangements have been made for you to tell your story to interrogating officers who will then ask you to write it down.

When we were children, our father never spoke about what had happened during the war, and our mother told us not to ask any questions. I recently learned that the troops were specifically ordered not to talk about their incarceration – the war was over and people at home did not want to hear any more tales of suffering. Louise Cordingly's[2] Echoes of Captivity found that many former Japanese POWs had immense difficulties settling back into civilian life. Several were psychologically damaged, having nightmares and flashbacks which affected their families, causing long-term problems, but this was not our experience. Harry was a cheerful, optimistic man, and it truly did not seem as if his time in captivity had affected him. All we knew was that he had eaten a lot of rice, suffered from recurring bouts of malaria and, typical of his rather wacky sense of humour, had a girlfriend called One Lung Too Few!

In the 1980s, our parents took a holiday in the Far East which included a couple of days in Singapore. They had arranged in advance to have a tour of Changi Gaol (now a civilian prison) and this obviously had a cathartic effect as after their return, my father got down an old leather case to show me the memorabilia of his war years. I was fascinated to see not just diaries, but also drawings and paintings, photographs, newspaper cuttings, medals, letters, telegrams, Japanese money and a canvas roll containing his medical kit. It was a real treasure trove.

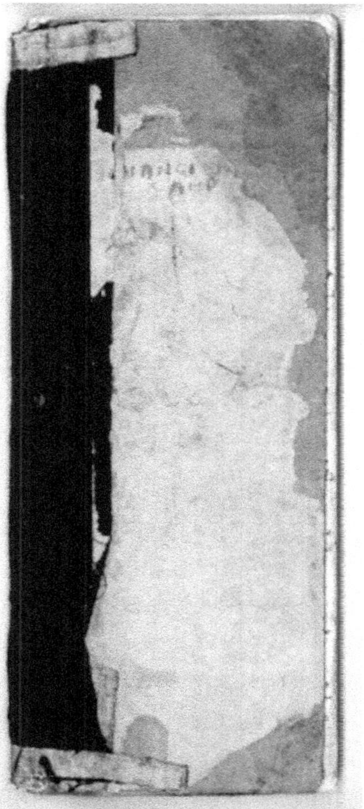

Cover of 4th Far East Diary

There is one small diary of his period in France at the outbreak of war, containing mainly memos and jottings. However, the four diaries of his time in the Far East contain detailed descriptions of capitulation and life as a prisoner of war of the Japanese. The first three were small three-month diaries, pharmaceutical give-aways. To begin with Harry wrote a daily entry on each page, but as he realised there would be a shortage of paper, his writing became smaller and smaller, and he wrote more fully only on days when he felt something of note had happened.

His supply of diaries ran out on Christmas Day 1942, but Harry was fortunate to find a partly-used bill of lading book in which he wrote in both pen and pencil. The paper was very thin, so to start with he only wrote on one side of the page. When he reached the end, he turned it over to write on the other side. This did not make the diary easy to read, particularly as his handwriting was a fairly typical doctor's scrawl. In addition, there were holes in several places where small sections had been deliberately cut out to eradicate evidence of an illegal radio, which was a death penalty offence.

To keep a diary at all was strictly forbidden. Harry concealed his in various places including under his mattress or sewn into his mattress. At one point when he was at a camp on the Burma Railway, he was given a sudden order to move, and did not have time to retrieve his diary. He was able to get a message to a friend who brought it up to him a week later.

Towards the end of his life Harry dictated to me sections of his diary which he thought would be of interest. I transcribed about a fifth of the diaries with his help and then completed the rest after his death. It was a shock for my sister, brother and me to find out what our father had actually been through, as he had made light of his wartime experiences, joking about the hardships and privations as if they were mere inconveniences. His diaries, an objective, articulate and occasionally humorous account of his time in captivity in the Far East, are now held in the Imperial War Museum.

Jim Bradley[5] sent my father a copy of his book, recounting his attempted escape from the Burma Railway. He enclosed a letter in which he wrote that he always felt that Harry was one of the great men in captivity.

For our family he was an amazing man who went out of his way to care for people throughout his life. He retained to the end both the compassion and sense of humour which we believe helped him to survive as a POW. It is my privilege to tell our father's story, as much as possible in his own words.

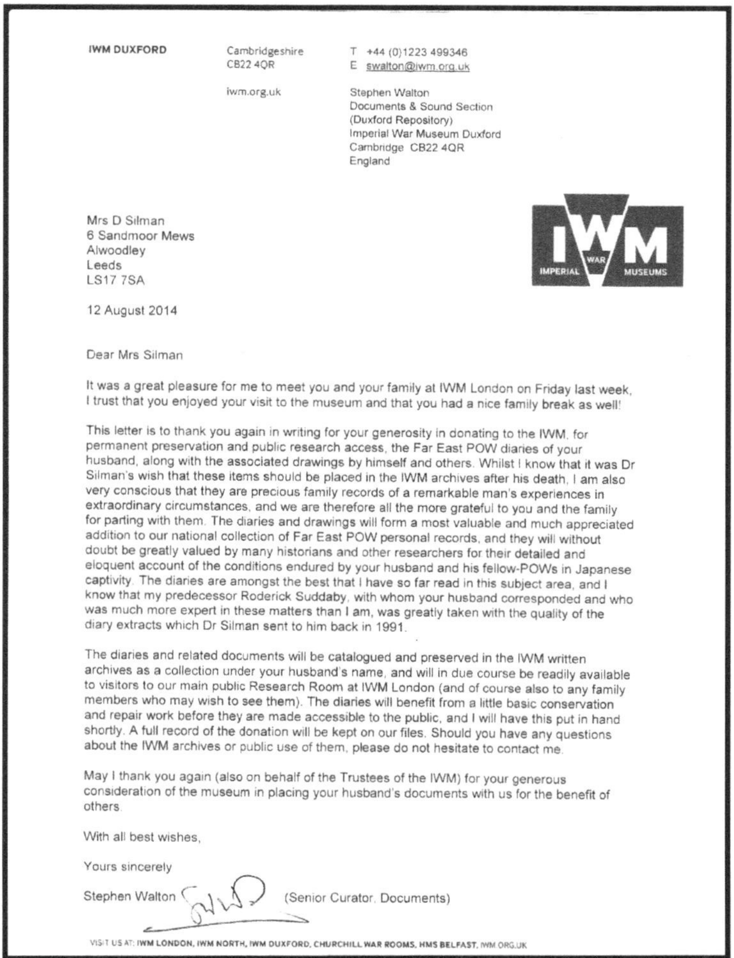

IWM DUXFORD

Cambridgeshire
CB22 4QR

iwm.org.uk

T +44 (0)1223 499346
E swalton@iwm.org.uk

Stephen Walton
Documents & Sound Section
(Duxford Repository)
Imperial War Museum Duxford
Cambridge CB22 4QR
England

IWM IMPERIAL WAR MUSEUMS

Mrs D Silman
6 Sandmoor Mews
Alwoodley
Leeds
LS17 7SA

12 August 2014

Dear Mrs Silman

It was a great pleasure for me to meet you and your family at IWM London on Friday last week. I trust that you enjoyed your visit to the museum and that you had a nice family break as well!

This letter is to thank you again in writing for your generosity in donating to the IWM, for permanent preservation and public research access, the Far East POW diaries of your husband, along with the associated drawings by himself and others. Whilst I know that it was Dr Silman's wish that these items should be placed in the IWM archives after his death, I am also very conscious that they are precious family records of a remarkable man's experiences in extraordinary circumstances, and we are therefore all the more grateful to you and the family for parting with them. The diaries and drawings will form a most valuable and much appreciated addition to our national collection of Far East POW personal records, and they will without doubt be greatly valued by many historians and other researchers for their detailed and eloquent account of the conditions endured by your husband and his fellow-POWs in Japanese captivity. The diaries are amongst the best that I have so far read in this subject area, and I know that my predecessor Roderick Suddaby, with whom your husband corresponded and who was much more expert in these matters than I am, was greatly taken with the quality of the diary extracts which Dr Silman sent to him back in 1991.

The diaries and related documents will be catalogued and preserved in the IWM written archives as a collection under your husband's name, and will in due course be readily available to visitors to our main public Research Room at IWM London (and of course also to any family members who may wish to see them). The diaries will benefit from a little basic conservation and repair work before they are made accessible to the public, and I will have this put in hand shortly. A full record of the donation will be kept on our files. Should you have any questions about the IWM archives or public use of them, please do not hesitate to contact me.

May I thank you again (also on behalf of the Trustees of the IWM) for your generous consideration of the museum in placing your husband's documents with us for the benefit of others.

With all best wishes,

Yours sincerely

Stephen Walton (Senior Curator, Documents)

VISIT US AT: IWM LONDON, IWM NORTH, IWM DUXFORD, CHURCHILL WAR ROOMS, HMS BELFAST, IWM.ORG.UK

Letter to Dorothea, Harry's widow, following transfer of Harry's war diaries and artworks to the Imperial War Museum

Chapter Two

Dunkirk

What a night! ... bombed, machine-gunned and shelled

Harry enlisted as soon as war was declared in September 1939, and was posted to the 9th Battalion, Royal Northumberland Fusiliers (RNF). He was told to report immediately so he set off in his old banger which broke down in Darlington. He continued by taxi to Newcastle but was upset to find that the reporting station did not yet exist, so he was put up in a hotel for three weeks. The battalion spent the winter training at Gosforth Park race course. They were woefully under-equipped. Although nominally a machine-gun battalion, they possessed only two machine guns which were German weapons captured in 1918.

The early days of the war became known as the 'phoney war' as there was virtually no combat. It gave the Allies time to train their troops in preparation for the battles that began when Germany invaded France in May 1940. The RNF, as part of the British Expeditionary Force (BEF), were sent to support the French.

They embarked on the SS Fenella at Southampton on St George's Day 23rd April 1940 – a significant day for the RNF as their emblem is St George and the Dragon. St George was to be a potent symbol for the RNF throughout the war. Padre Cordingly[4] named the chapels he consecrated in Singapore and Thailand after St George, and Fusilier George[6] chose it as his pseudonym. Even in captivity in Changi, they celebrated St George's Day: *23rd April 1942 St George's Day dawned bright & clear (& very hot). We all went home & made roses in our hats – made out of red flags & white bandages. Everyone appeared to have a sparkle in their eyes.*

The RNF had the task of constructing an airfield. The week was divided into four days working on the airfields, two days training and a day of rest. The official history of the RNF[7] states that 'as the role was a working and not a fighting one, the Division proceeded on a much-reduced scale of weapons, equipment and transport.' The two ancient

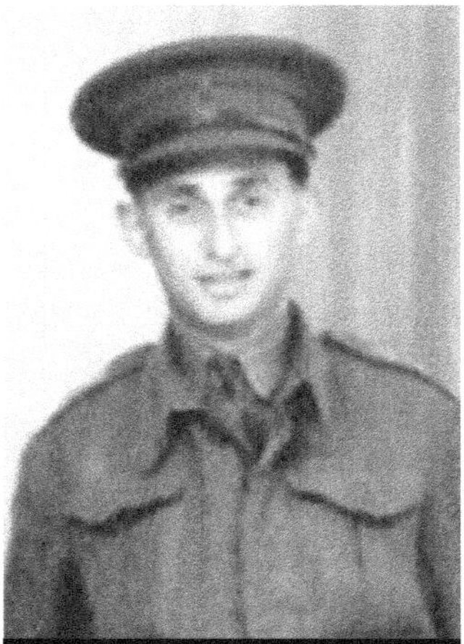
Captain Harry Silman

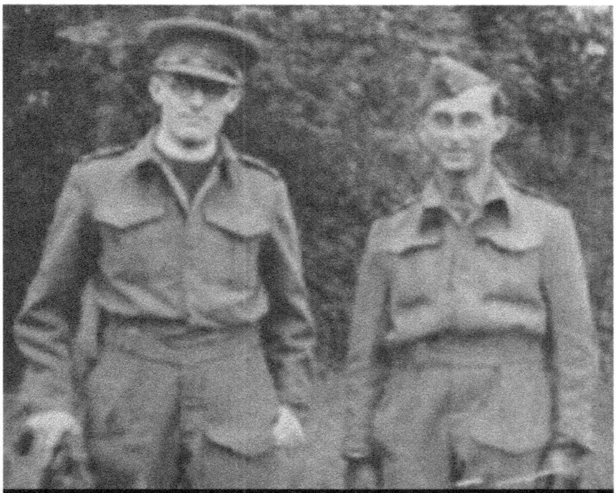
Harry and Padre Cordingly in northern France

machine guns were supplemented with a further 24, plus an anti-tank rifle – a 'skeleton scale of equipment'.

They stayed in various small towns and villages and were welcomed by the French. Fusilier George[6] wrote 'Many and frequent were the bottles of wine that were cracked in celebration of our arrival to the furthering of the Entente Cordiale and to the speedy and utter downfall of the Hun.' It was a holiday atmosphere and the army put on variety concerts as entertainment. There were only a few minor medical problems requiring Harry's attention such as a fractured hand, bronchitis, pneumonia, scabies, a query appendicitis and two *fake cases*.

After living under canvas since arriving in France, Harry was billeted in a chateau in Lillers, a small farming town 15 km west of Béthune. There were constant air raid sirens which were generally ignored. *The weather has kept very fine and sunny for the past two weeks and life is very pleasant. I am now sitting in the garden behind the Chateau in the hot sunshine with a Sapper book on one side, some chocolate on the other side and my writing pad on my knee.*

This almost idyllic rural existence ended abruptly when the German offensive began. 'Friday 10th May 1940 will surely go down through the ages as one of the milestones of History. We were all awakened at about 0400 hours by the sound of heavy gunfire and the drone of internal combustion engines. The sky was dotted with small puffs of white smoke and there were to be seen a number of aircraft obviously of Hun extraction'.[6]

For the next few days, the battalion went into defensive mode in fear of a parachute landing. The division was moved to the right flank of the BEF in case of an unexpected German advance. They were spread out into neighbouring towns, but all the roads were clogged with refugees. The British troops then moved steadily northwards to reach Steenbecque where they had the most intense combat of the war to date, defending the ridge which was surrounded by German tanks. *Went into action against German tanks. We looked like being overwhelmed – troop carriers are reported to have landed. No sleep for 3 nights, must have affected the lads. Who can defend themselves against tanks with rifles? Where is the air force?*

Major General Curtis sent the 9th RNF a congratulatory telegram the next day saying that if they had not held the Steenbecque Ridge against tanks and infantry, the Boches might now be in Dunkirk.

They were then ordered to withdraw, and retreated to Dunkirk under constant bombardment. On 29th May, Harry made a brief diary entry: *What a night! Travelling in the rain, bombed, machine-gunned and shelled. Hear that British army is evacuating this sector. Anticipate terrible slaughter on roads.*

It was total chaos on the beaches, so Harry took over a local café for his patients. There he delivered three babies to local women. He commandeered a truck to transport the sick and injured over the sand to the waiting boats. This was a difficult task as apart from the constant bombing, he had to swerve frequently to avoid soldiers who, while they were waiting, part-buried themselves in the sand for protection,

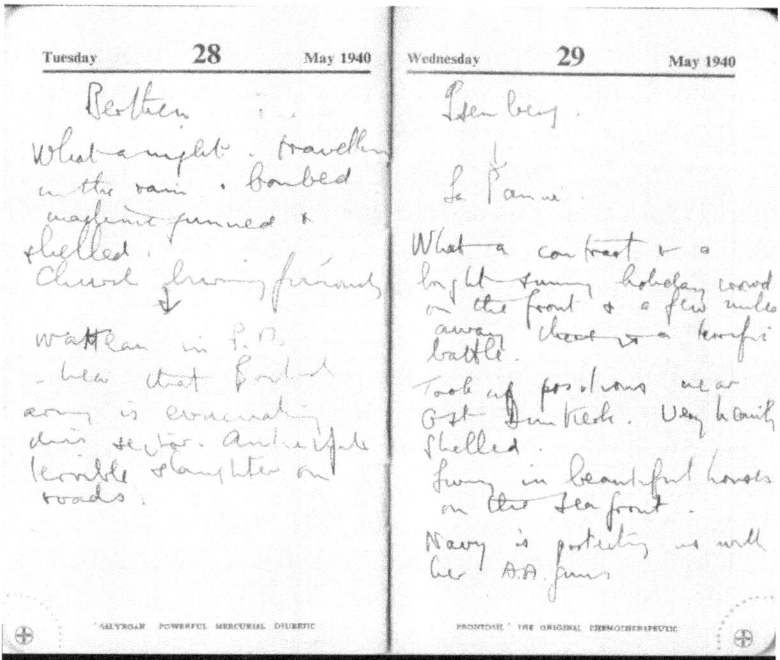
Tuesday 28 May 1940

Berthen

What a night. travelling in the rain. bombed machine gunned & shelled.
Church burning furiously
↓
Watteau in P.B.
- hear that French army is evacuating this sector. And the terrible slaughter on roads.

Wednesday 29 May 1940

Steenbecq.
↓
La Panne.

What a contrast - a bright sunny holiday crowd on the front & a few miles away there is a terrific battle.
Took up positions near Ost Dunkerk. Very heavily shelled.
Living in beautiful houses on the sea front.
Navy is protecting us with his A.A. guns

SALYRGAN POWERFUL MERCURIAL DIURETIC

PRONTOSIL THE ORIGINAL CHEMOTHERAPEUTIC

Extract from Dunkirk Diary

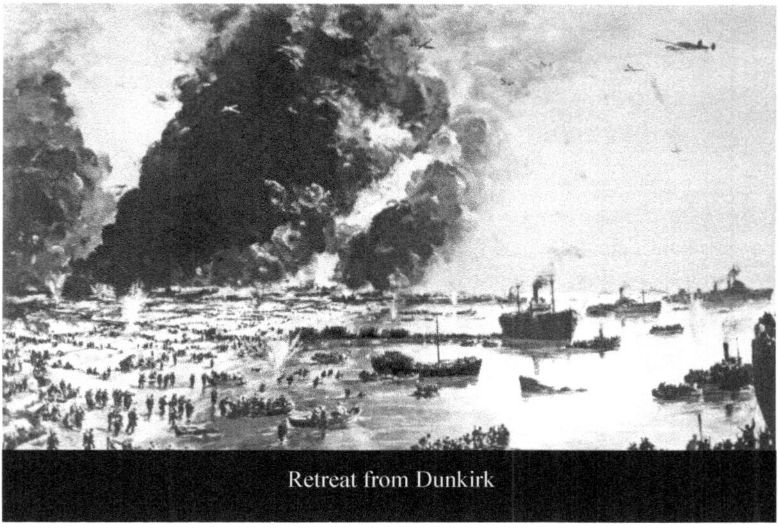
Retreat from Dunkirk

with only their heads showing. In a letter to his elder brother four days later, he wrote: *I could hear the shells and bombs bursting all around. It was a nightmare ride that I shall not forget in a hurry.*

He made several journeys before he ran out of fuel, and walked the last stretch. He got away on the destroyer HMS *Malcolm*, accompanying the wounded he had rescued. A letter written by Montague Burton[8] to Harry's father praises Harry's 'bravery, self-possession and calmness in the firing-line'.

During the period between the retreat at Dunkirk in June 1940 and departure for the eventual destination of Singapore in October 1941, the battalion was strengthened, properly equipped and trained in the UK. They were deployed first to defend the coastline in Devon and then Norfolk, waiting for a German invasion which did not materialise. They had further training in Scotland, Cheshire, Wiltshire and North Wales. By the end of this the 18th Division 'had become a highly-trained formation, and the RNF a first-class machine gun unit.'[7]

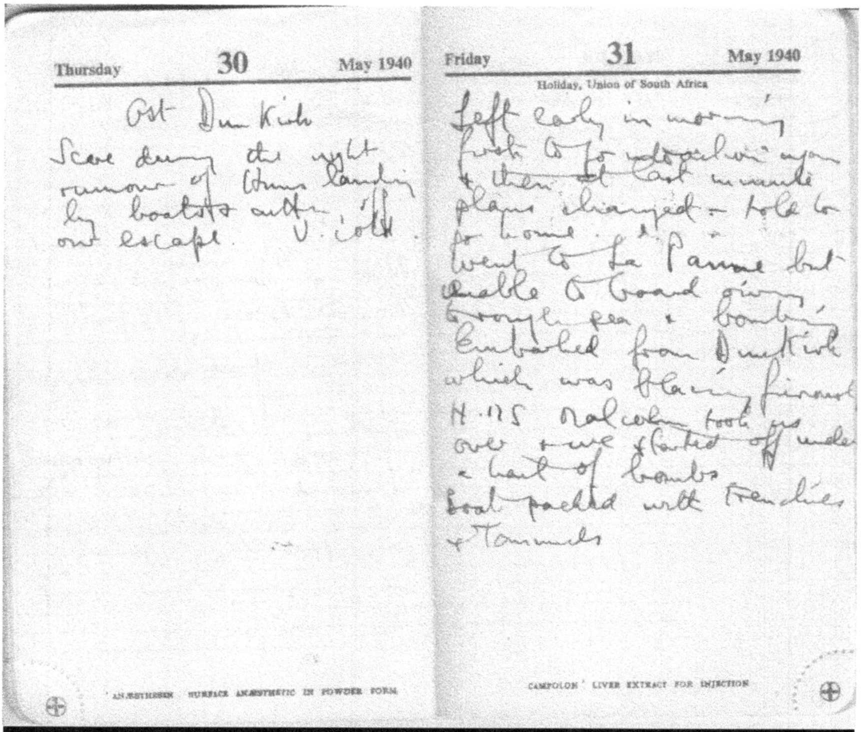
Thursday 30 May 1940

Ost Dunkirk

Scare during the night
rumour of Huns landing
by boats to cut off
our escape. V. cold.

ANÆSTHESIN SURFACE ANÆSTHETIC IN POWDER FORM

Friday 31 May 1940

Holiday, Union of South Africa

Left early in morning
for [illegible] again
+ then at last minute
plans changed – told to
go home.
Went to La Panne but
unable to board owing
to rough sea + bombing.
Embarked from Dunkirk
which was blazing fiercely
H.M.S. Malcolm took us
over + we started off under
a hail of bombs
Boat packed with Frenchies
+ Tommies

CAMPOLON LIVER EXTRACT FOR INJECTION

Extract from Dunkirk Diary

Chapter Three

Singapore

Arrived at Singapore after an exciting morning with the Jap bombers

Part of the battalion embarked in Greenock on 27th October 1941 and the rest of the 18th Division were picked up from Liverpool and Avonmouth two days later. Their planned destination was debatable as the men were not given this information. Harry and Padre Cordingly thought they were bound for Egypt while Jim Bradley[5] wrote that the most informed rumour was that they were heading for the Persian Gulf, with the object of linking up with the Russians in the Caucasus.

The British *Warwick Castle* was their first ship on the journey, taking them to Halifax in Nova Scotia. It was a roundabout route to avoid sailing near the European front. From Halifax they followed the coast of Canada and eastern USA on the American *Orizaba*, protected by the United States navy. At this time, America was not involved in the war, but there was an agreement that they would escort British troop carriers. From there they sailed to Trinidad and arrived into Cape Town on 9th December.

Crucially on 7th December, two days before Harry arrived in South Africa, the Japanese attacked Pearl Harbour, the US naval base in Hawaii. This had the immediate effect of bringing the USA into the war. What is often forgotten is that the Japanese also attacked, on that same day, the British base in Hong Kong and the RAF bases on the coast of Malaya to the north of Singapore, ensuring that the RAF would neither be able to retaliate, nor protect their own troops. Britain declared war on Japan on December 8th and on December 10th the Japanese torpedoed the *Prince of Wales* and the *Repulse* which were at the head of the fleet of ships sent to defend the island of Singapore.

The sudden Japanese attack resulted in the 18th Division being diverted to defend the British military base in Singapore. They went via Mombasa to a camp at Deolali near Bombay. They had set out

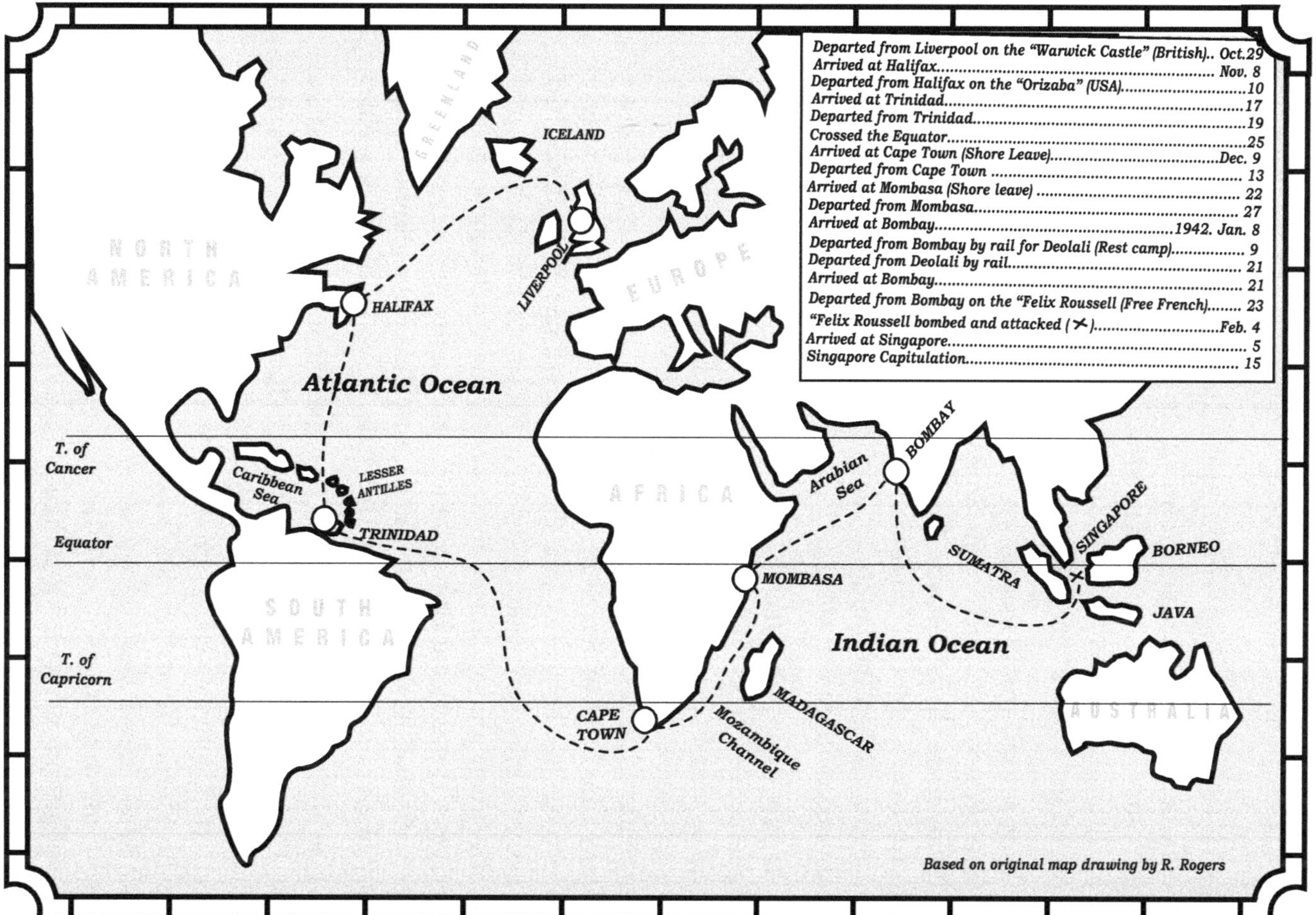

Route to Singapore 29 Oct 1941 – 5 Feb 1942

prepared for desert fighting, with no provision for tropical conditions. In Deolali they had a fortnight's training, acclimatising and checking transport and equipment, but there were no inoculations against tropical diseases such as malaria. In reality, the troops were totally unequipped for a war in the Far East.

They set sail from Bombay on 23rd January 1942 on the French ship *Felix Roussel* and arrived in Singapore on 5th February, which was already under heavy bombardment by the Japanese. The freighter which was carrying the battalion's transport did not manage to unload before it fled the bombing, so the RNF had to make do with requisitioned civilian vehicles.

At the time, the island of Singapore was thought to be impregnable, a fortress able to withstand any sea or air attack. To this end, there were huge gun fortifications which pointed out south to sea for the suspected invasion. The British newsreels and Churchill had engendered a general confidence that the British could protect Singapore, the 'city of the lion', as it was one of the most strongly fortified bases in the world, and the many civilians living there had been assured they were safe. However, with both the air force and navy effectively out of action, it was easy for the Japanese to take advantage of the arrogant British belief that Singapore was invincible, and they attacked from the north via the so-called impenetrable jungle – a way of entry dismissed by the British as being highly improbable.

It is also possible that British HQ knew that they were sending the 18th Division to a lost cause, but it was judged politically expedient that the Australian troops were not left to defend the island without support. In his diary, Harry reports on a talk by Major General Beckwith-Smith. *He praised the men for their part in that action on the island & hoped that we would soon show our true worth. Our coming to the island was a political & not a military fault.* It was a sacrificial gesture which led to a dreadful waste of life.

When the Division first arrived on the island, apart from the noise of the shelling there was none of the atmosphere of the war-torn Britain they had left behind, with its blackouts and curfews. Bill Frankland[9] said it did not seem like war at all, as all the lights were on and the city sparkled at night.

Although the troops were under a Japanese barrage, they still had freedom of movement. *I was able to take some very interesting films during the battle and the immediate aftermath. I was very careful with the camera and the films. I sewed the camera and the films up in a canvas bag, and I decided to hide it somewhere until the end of the war. The padre took over a little mosque, next door to our billet. I climbed into the roof of the mosque into a circular dome. I pushed the camera and films into a very dark recess and I hope to reclaim them after the war.* Before he went up country, Harry checked everything was there. *Unfortunately, I found that someone had stolen it all. How someone knew it was there, or how it was spotted in the darkness, I do not know. Well that is that. I mourn the loss of the films more than the camera. The former are irreplaceable.*

Singapore was virtually lost by the time the 18th Division arrived on 5th February 1942. They slept the first night on damp grass with no shelter. The next night Harry shared a tent with the Padre, Eric Cordingly. Their friendship had started in France and continued throughout their captivity in the Far East.

The first ten days were spent collecting supplies and setting up medical arrangements including a field ambulance. *9th February: News received that the Japanese had effected a landing on the west coast and were advancing. This part of the coast had been defended by 'West Force' composed mainly of Australians who had fought on the mainland. They did not appear to offer much resistance to the landing forces. Consequently the Japs were able to land large forces without much hindrance and advanced eastward. The advance was preceded by a terrific barrage which we heard in the early hours of the morning and sounded like a continuous rumble.*

They alternated between sleeping under canvas and in houses which had been deserted by the civilian population. *Friday 13th February: We had a morning of scares and shelling but managed to get a good breakfast served in the house which served as the mess. Had a wash & shave in the bathroom – a luxury – and helped myself to some clothing and underwear – justifiable looting in wartime.*

It seems scarcely believable that during the period before surrender, the officers arranged a ball at Raffles Hotel. A photograph was taken of them in their dress uniform, and it was hanging in Raffles Hotel when my parents visited Singapore in the late 80s.

Chapter Four

Surrender

Sunday 15th February 1942: Very momentous day

Much has been written about the fall of Singapore, with most historians and military analysts in agreement that we lost Singapore owing to several catastrophic mistakes. In December 1942, General Percival published an article in the local Syonan Times on 'Why We Were Defeated' and Harry commented: *Percival says plainly that our troops were unseasoned, couldn't fight for long periods, lack of air support & absence of coastal defences on the north shore of Singapore. He also mentions the speed of the Jap advance which probably was too fast for our slowly moving army minds.* Churchill admitted it was the worst disaster and largest capitulation in British history.

One of the most horrific atrocities during this period was the brutal massacre of the medical staff and patients at the Alexandra Hospital. On 14th February, the hospital was under attack. A British medical officer wearing a Red Cross armband came out but was fired at. As he ran back he was followed by the Japanese soldiers who went from ward to ward, shooting, bayoneting or beating doctors, nurses and patients indiscriminately, including killing an anaesthetised patient who was waiting for an operation. Those who were not murdered in the hospital were either killed as they fled, or rounded up and executed the following morning. In the post-war Japanese war crime trials, there was no evidence to prove the identity of the main perpetrators, and they were never brought to justice.

Although the British troops could clearly see the signs of what was to come, Harry's diary entry for 14th February is still fairly relaxed in spite of the severity of the attack around him: *Very busy day for me as the casualties came pouring in and the ambulance I had picked up was a godsend. The Padre stayed in the RAP and did good work cheering up the wounded. We buried one man behind our tent. Intense mortar fire made us crouch down most of the day and our tent was ripped by shrapnel many times. Meals in the mess were interrupted by bombing and a lovely evening meal was spoiled as we had to take cover for over an hour – being dark when we returned. Decided to get a good night's rest so slept in bed with sheets!*

By the next day it was all over. *Very momentous day. In morning had a good deal of attention from planes, guns and mortars and started to dig a deeper trench in the southern pit of the RAP. Numerous casualties including about 8 shell shock cases – the latter were packed off into the deep shelter. The ambulance worked splendidly getting the wounded away and the driver did very good work dodging shells and shell holes.*

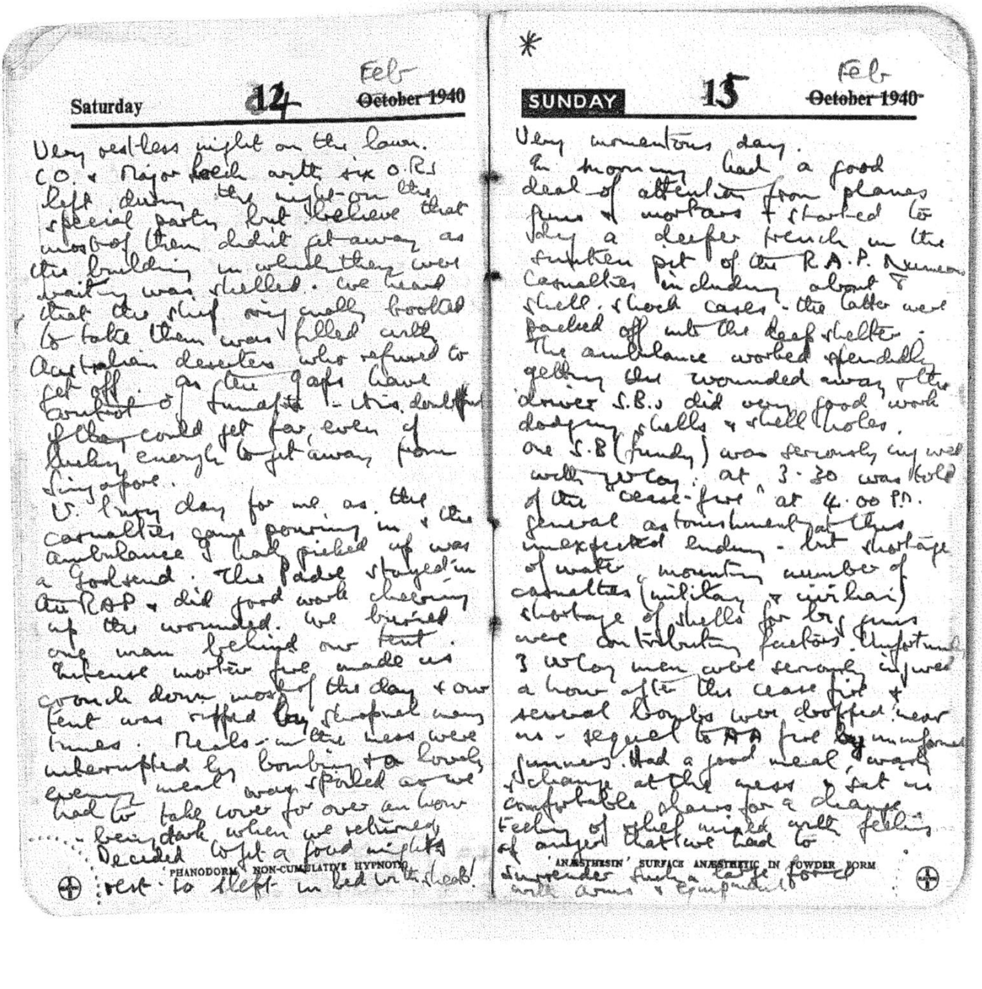

Saturday 14 ~~October 1940~~ Feb

Very restless night on the lawn. C.O. & Major [illegible] with six O.Rs left during the night on the special party but believe that most of them didn't get away as the building in which they were waiting was shelled. We heard that the ship originally booked to take them was filled with Australian deserters who refused to get off as the Japs have control of [illegible] – this doubtful if they could get far, even if lucky enough to get away from Singapore.
V. busy day for me as the casualties came pouring in & the ambulance I had picked up was a Godsend. The Padre stayed in the RAP & did good work cheering up the wounded. We buried one man behind our tent. Intense mortar fire made us crouch down most of the day & our tent was ripped by shrapnel many times. Meals in the mess were interrupted by bombing & a lovely evening meal was spoiled as we had to take cover for over an hour – being dark when we returned. Decided to get a good night's rest so slept in bed with sheets!

PHANODORM NON-CUMULATIVE HYPNOTIC

SUNDAY 15 ~~October 1940~~ Feb

Very momentous day. In morning had a good deal of attention from planes guns & mortars & started to dig a deeper trench in the southern pit of the R.A.P. Numerous casualties including about 8 shell shock cases – the latter were packed off into the deep shelter. The ambulance worked splendidly getting the wounded away & the driver S.B.s did very good work dodging shells & shell holes. One S.B. ([illegible]) was seriously injured with [illegible]. At 3.30 was told of the "cease-fire" at 4.00 PM. General astonishment at this unexpected ending – but shortage of water, mounting number of casualties (military & civilian), shortage of shells for [illegible] guns were contributing factors. Unfortunately 3 [illegible] men were seriously injured a hour after the cease fire & several bombs were dropped near us – sequel to AA fire by uninformed gunners. Had a good meal & a change at the mess & sat in comfortable chairs for a change. Feeling of relief mixed with feelings of anger that we had to surrender such a large force with arms & equipment.

ANÆSTHESIN SURFACE ANÆSTHETIC IN POWDER FORM

General Percival took the decision to surrender. It is clear from Harry's diary that this was not anticipated: *At 3.30 was told of the "ceasefire" at 4.00pm. General astonishment at this unexpected ending – but shortage of water, mounting number of casualties (military and civilian), shortage of shells for big guns were contributing factors. Unfortunately 3 W Company men were seriously injured an hour after the ceasefire and several bombs were dropped near us – sequel to AA fire by uninformed gunners. Had a good meal, wash and change at the mess and sat on comfortable chairs for a change. Feeling of relief mixed with feeling of anger that we had to surrender such a large force with arms and equipment.*

The Padre shared this feeling[4]: 'It had been a nine-day wonder and while it lasted, tense and exciting, but in reality rather more tragic and shattering. There was greatness in sacrifice and service, but war waged with modern weapons can have no glamour… We should not have been forced to lay down our arms, but the decision was not ours'.

The day following surrender, Harry went behind the Japanese lines with the Padre and a burial party to collect the casualties from the heavy bombing: *16 Feb Very difficult job as the bodies were swollen black and sizzling in the heat. The men in the Bren carriers were mangled and burnt, making identification impossible.*

Approximately 100,000 British, Australian and Indian troops were marched 17 miles to Changi, a former British military base in the north-east of Singapore island to begin their captivity as prisoners of war.

Chapter Five

Changi

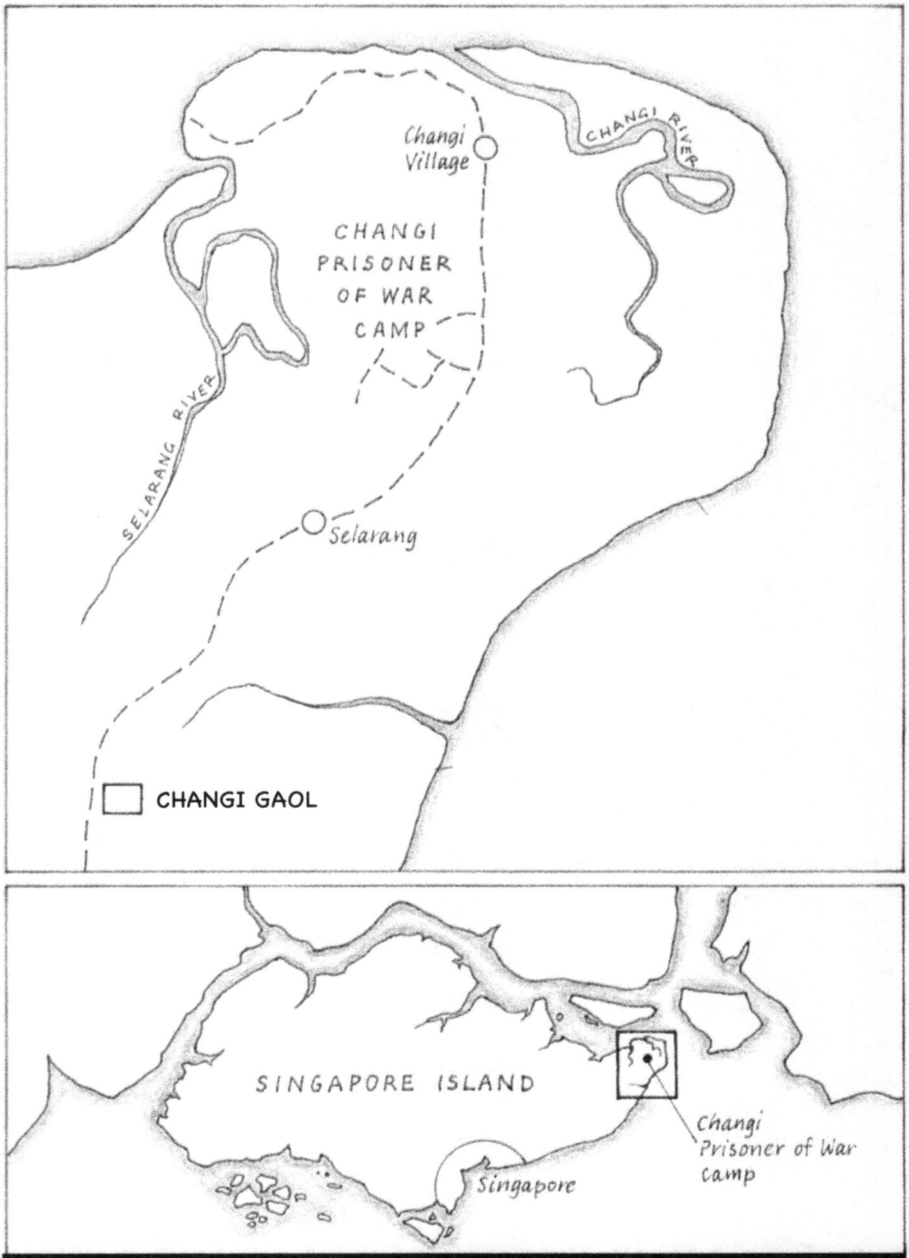

Location of Changi POW camp, Selarang and Changi Gaol from maps drawn by David Cordingly

My days are settling down

Changi lies in the north-east of Singapore close to the Equator. It is always hot and humid, with heavy monsoon rains for approximately six months of the year and no real dry season. Today there are wide roads leading to Changi airport. In the early 1940s the ground was swampy with exceptionally dense vegetation of palm and rubber trees, making any escape attempt fraught with hazard.

A communiqué with a list of rules and prohibitions was issued by the Japanese High Command on the day following surrender. These included a total ban on all wireless communication and any contact with the outside world. This did not stop the POWs, who listened to illegal radios in secret, getting up-to-date news of the war in Europe. Radio components were hidden in the hollow bamboo chair legs and sink pipes of Harry's MI room. However, this involved great risk, punishable by death, and every so often he cut out tiny sections of the diary which would have indicated to the Japanese that he had access to an illicit radio.

The sewage system, water supply and electric lighting had all been destroyed, so rectifying these problems took precedence: *The electric light plant was taken from a large house outside the wire, & brought in by a party of RAOC chaps who fitted it up themselves. They have done an excellent job... giving us light which is on from 8.15 – 10.45. The Japs now know about it and have cast covetous eyes on it, so that if they think they may require it, they may whip it all away.*

Sanitary arrangements were non-existent at first. There was a major dysentery epidemic which affected 40% of the prison population within three days of their arrival. At the time there was little understanding among the troops of the importance of hygiene. They had to dig latrines as quickly as possible and build anti-malarial drains. *The latrines are now working, but being Indian style it is rather uncomfortable till one gets used to it. Still it is a relief not to have hundreds of bluebottles biting one's bottom.*

Until the engineers got a proper water system going, each man was rationed to four pints of water per person a day for all purposes. This water was from a water cart and not pure, so before they could drink it, it had to be chlorinated.

After the shock of finding a convalescing dysentery patient cleaning dixies in the cookhouse, Harry took on the responsibility for educating the cookhouse workers about the necessity for hygiene and the safe method of cooking rice. *As part of the blitz against dysentery, all mess tins etc have to be dipped in boiling water and sterilised before and after meals.*

He then started a series of lectures to all the troops on dysentery, fly measures, skin disease, vitamins and general hygiene with posters to help. He was rather nervous at first as it had been a long time since he addressed a gathering, but after the first five minutes, he regained his old confidence. *Fly propaganda is going on nicely, & all men have been lectured, & numerous gruesome placards adorn cookhouses & billets. 25 deaths in the past 4 days is a high mortality rate, and all measures possible must be adopted. Very annoyed with W & Z companies for having lukewarm water for sterilising, after all my efforts. We still meet chaos in some depts., eg the swill, – in spite of the order that swill should be burnt in the incinerator, they sent the stuff back to put on the garden!* He persevered and eventually completed lectures to all the Companies.

The accommodation in Changi was totally inadequate for the number of troops imprisoned there. They quickly erected bamboo-framed huts covered with canvas, tarpaulins or anything that was suitable. After a short time, part of the 18th Division were allocated to the former India Lines. They were given two barrack blocks, one for the officers – *we cleaned up the billet & divided it into three: (i) library (ii) sleeping (iii) ante-room. There are several armchairs & tables available & numerous old newspapers so that it resembles old times again* – and the second for senior NCOs. These blocks were originally intended to house 150, but now housed between 600-800.

The junior NCOs and troops were given wooden huts and tents, so everyone had protection from the rain which was unlike any rainfall they had experienced in England. In the monsoon season, the rain was torrential, completely drenching clothing and equipment, and tearing down trees and wires. However the rain did have advantages: *Occasional showers are welcomed as we take off our clothing and taking a piece of soap, step out into the rain and give ourselves a good clean up.*

Changi had originally been a large British military base which had been hastily evacuated on 7th February. It had suffered from looting by the time it was turned into a POW camp, but there were many odd materials lying around which were put to good use. *By begging, scrounging and borrowing, have managed to collect a reasonable amount of personal kit which I have stowed away in my locker and have borrowed a blanket to cover my sofa-cushion, which on a table top serves as my bed. Found a camp chair and a small wooden table so am quite comfortable for the time being.*

The prisoners were short of basic items of clothing and equipment. Harry had overcome his scruples in taking items from deserted homes in Singapore Town, but he noted these in his diary and intended to apologise to 'Mr Reeves' after the war.

List of my Personal Possessions and their former or present owners

Wristlet watch	*Loaned by Archie*
Blanket	*Loaned by Eva*
Pillow case	*Given by Addy*
Shoes *Topee* *Towel* *ARP raincoat* *Hankies* *Blue shorts*	*Borrowed from Mr Reeves of Singapore (without his knowledge or permission)*
Coloured shirt	*Given by Thornhill*
Short pants	*Taken from some house in Singapore*
2 pairs stockings	*CO's kit left behind*
2 pairs KD shorts *2 K shirts*	*Taken from Singapore laundry*
1 stick	*Converted golf club*
1 Forage cap	*Made by me from battle dress trousers of Webb*
1 pair slippers	*Made from old tyres*
1 haversack	*Given by Macreath*
1 spring bed	*Supplied by hospital*
1 long sofa cushion (used as mattress)	*Mr Reeves*
Mosquito net	*"Found"*
1 folding camp chair	*"Found"*
1 table	*"Found"*

In June 1942, the Imperial Japanese Army started to pay the POWs an amenity grant: *The amazing part is that the Japs are printing unnumbered notes & giving them to us as an amenity grant, & we are buying the stores which were left behind by the British or were looted from stores. The whole position is ludicrous. It is difficult to ascertain who is making a profit out of these transactions.* Later, thanks to the personal intervention of the General, they were paid on a more official footing. The Changi guards told them they were very fortunate to get paid, as the rule was no work, no pay. POWs in other Japanese prison camps received no pay at all unless they were doing hard labour.

The money helped them to buy extra supplies from the natives who ran a lucrative business selling back to the soldiers *all the cigarette and food stores they stole from the barracks. This has to be done surreptitiously as the Japs would shoot both the vendor and emptor if they saw the transactions.* The funds also enabled them to buy basic necessities: *More canteen stores have arrived. I just managed to scrape together sufficient money to pay for some shaving cream, a tooth brush, boot polish etc.*

They received infrequent supplies from contacts in Singapore Town who boxed up random items they were able to acquire. Occasionally there was disappointment when the packages were opened: *When we opened Henry's box from S. which had been packed ready for dispatch for the past 3 months, it was found that the packets of fruit pastilles had melted & mixed with the soap, sugar & toothpaste to form a conglomerate sticky mass. However much of the contents were rescued, but what we are to do with the enormous quantity of soap is not yet decided. I am trying to exchange some of it for bread which an officer is trying to sell.*

After about 4 months they were allowed to send one censored postcard home: *Many of the postcards have been returned as the writing is illegible & the senders have broken rules. In future it will be limited to 24 words clearly written. Wrote the postcard home in block letters, being very careful not to include double meanings, Braille etc. Simple childish sentences were the order of the day – I wonder what they will think at home when they see my effort. Still the main thing is to get some sort of message home telling them that I am fit.*

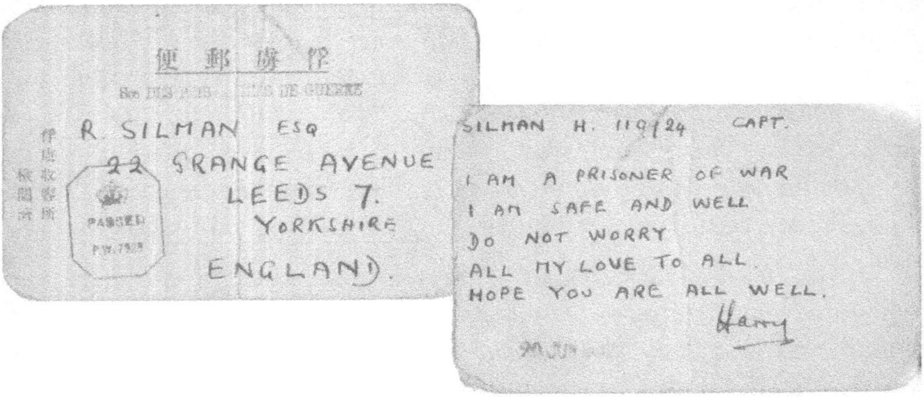

R. SILMAN ESQ
22 GRANGE AVENUE
LEEDS 7.
YORKSHIRE
ENGLAND.

SILMAN H. 119/24 CAPT.
I AM A PRISONER OF WAR
I AM SAFE AND WELL
DO NOT WORRY
ALL MY LOVE TO ALL
HOPE YOU ARE ALL WELL.
Harry

Harry's postcard dropped through the letterbox, but unfortunately it slid under a rug, and was not found until nearly six months later. It was 17th December (ten months after he was captured) before the family knew for certain that he was alive.

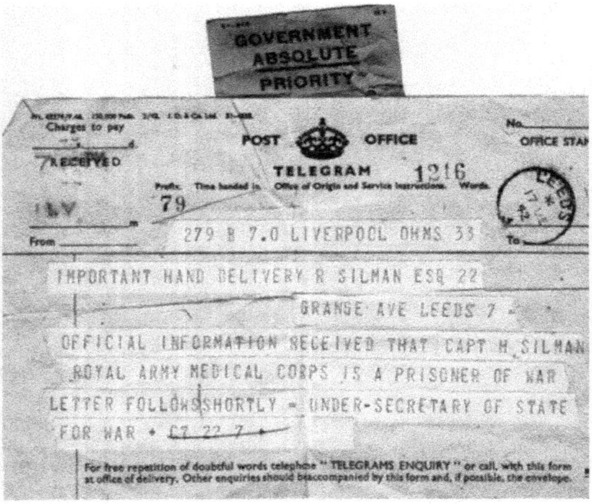

GOVERNMENT ABSOLUTE PRIORITY

POST OFFICE
TELEGRAM
1216
79
279 B 7.0 LIVERPOOL OHMS 33
IMPORTANT HAND DELIVERY R SILMAN ESQ 22
GRANGE AVE LEEDS 7 -
OFFICIAL INFORMATION RECEIVED THAT CAPT H SILMAN
ROYAL ARMY MEDICAL CORPS IS A PRISONER OF WAR
LETTER FOLLOWS SHORTLY - UNDER-SECRETARY OF STATE
FOR WAR • C7 22 7 •

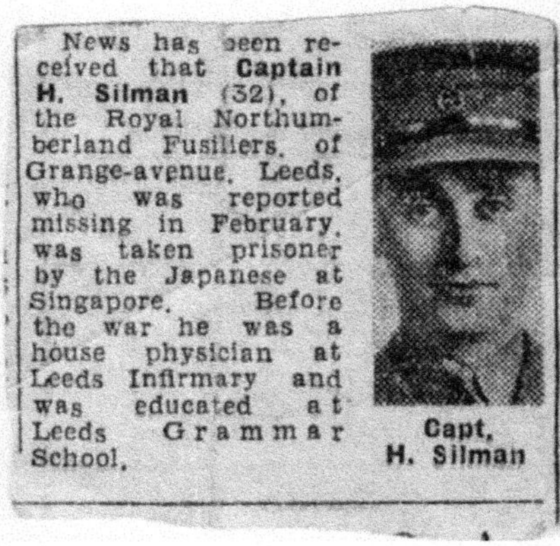

News has been received that **Captain H. Silman** (32), of the Royal Northumberland Fusiliers, of Grange-avenue, Leeds, who was reported missing in February, was taken prisoner by the Japanese at Singapore. Before the war he was a house physician at Leeds Infirmary and was educated at Leeds Grammar School.

Capt. H. Silman

There were sporadic grumbles about those in authority. However, a universally beloved figure was Major General Beckwith-Smith who died of heart failure, possibly following diphtheria, after being sent from Changi to Formosa. Harry said the news of Becky's death was a terrible blow to everyone in the 18th Division as he was very much respected and loved. *We all hoped that when we got back to England, he would act as our spokesman & explain the raw deal that our Div got in this battle.* Even the local Japanese propaganda newspaper, the Syonan Times, gave a front-page column to his death describing the homage that was paid to him as he lay in state by Japanese and Allied Commanders alike.

Harry occasionally came across people he knew or with whom he shared mutual acquaintances. Maybe the strangest coincidence was the man who was at sick parade one morning: *He told me where I live, & complained about the large postal packets I used to get. He was our postman. What a small world!*

Even in these early months, there were regular reminders of the cruelty of their captors: *Burn had a bad time to start with, as he was put in a barbed wire cage with no protection against the elements...The Japs have chopped off the hands of several Chinese & Malayans & decorating them with ribbons have hung them up in public places as a warning to looters & rioters. This puts the clock back several hundred years.*

Harry was also concerned that cultural differences could lead to punishment. *Three Jap guards came into the mess during the morning & I had to entertain them with tea & biscuits. Their knowledge of English was confined to Thank you, and we were thanking each other very often. They were amiable, and except for throwing the tea dregs on the floor, behaved very well. They offered me a cigarette & when I refused they started mumbling to each other – I wondered whether I had insulted them.*

*

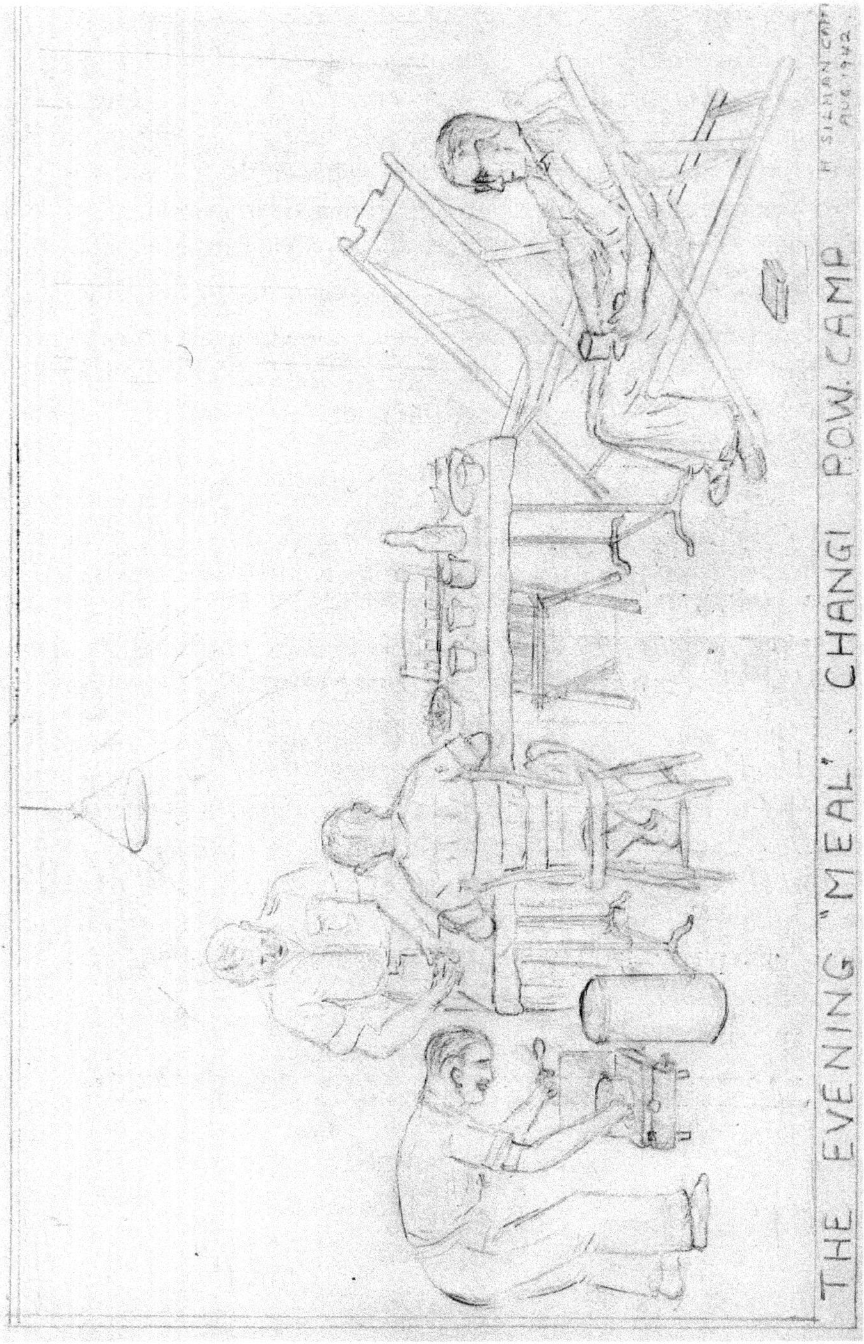
THE EVENING "MEAL". CHANGI P.O.W. CAMP
H SILMAN CAPT
AUG 1942

The food question is rather important

Food was a major concern and meals were eagerly anticipated, not just because the men were desperately hungry but also to break up the monotony of the day. It is understandable that Harry frequently writes about food in his diaries. After a few months he said he was getting used to the short rations and had lost that continual sense of slight hunger, but he was definitely below par in general fitness.

To begin with, the meals consisted almost entirely of their army rations of bully beef (tinned corn beef) and hardtack biscuits (a type of cracker): *The food is causing many grumbles as the midday meal consists of tea and three biscuits and there is nothing till 6.30 when we partake of a bully beef stew and more tea and biscuits. Tea is served without milk or sugar – soon it will be without tea.*

The staple food was rice, and in the early days this was virtually all they had: *We are getting almost ¾ lb of rice a day in various forms but mostly boiled – sometimes curried and sometimes with stew. Some of the meals consist of sugarless tea and tasteless rice – causing discontent. The cooks are being changed in the hope of getting tastier meals. There is too much eyeing the other fellows' rations and the complaints about other units getting more or better rations are numerous and groundless. There is a mad scramble after the meals have been issued for the small quantity left over in the dixies. It amazes me how the men can consume such large quantities of rice by itself. They can't possibly be hungry after a meal. I'm full of rice but the chaps come back for more.* After a new messing officer was appointed, the food started to improve and there were fewer complaints.

Whenever the Japanese wanted to punish the prisoners, the food was restricted to just rice: *A soldier from Southern Command was found outside the wire two nights ago and was shot by the Japs. They have punished us all by stopping our next meat, cigarette and soap ration. We will have to live almost on rice alone for the next week.*

The cooks became quite inventive with rice. The very popular breakfast porridge was made with ground rice and sweetened with diluted condensed milk. Harry said he felt comfortable and happy after breakfast which would set him up for the day. His batman roasted some rice grains which Harry ground into a powder and stirred into boiling water and declared it tasted like good coffee.

They were able to get supplies of meat from Singapore Town but they had occasional problems. *The large supply of fresh meat went bad today and we will have two meatless days. It was sheer stupidity keeping that meat in lukewarm water overnight. We have to be very careful of every morsel of protein and vitamin… Half the meat supply to the camp was condemned as being bad – this was due to the refrigerator in Singapore going off. The meat should have been used up quickly – it was a heart-breaking sight to see all the carcasses being buried and men eating plain rice. The diet is bound to have an effect on the general health and teeth in the long run.*

They also kept chickens and ducks with varying degrees of success: *The officers' mess bought 20 chickens locally and are keeping them in a hastily erected hen run at the back.* Then, two days later: *Chickens bought for the mess are dying off rapidly maybe due to croup. It is possible that the Malayans, finding the disease spreading among a brood, sell the seemingly healthy ones off cheaply and after the incubation period of the disease the birds die.* They could buy eggs from the Local Purchase Canteen but they were in short supply. *It is about 4 months since I last tasted an egg – one of the dishes that I really miss.*

They sometimes had quite remarkably good meals considering their incarceration: *The combined efforts of the MOs caused the deaths of ten of the ducks for dinner tonight – a good portion for each officer with roast potatoes, veg & stuffing, followed by a doughnut & cream!*

The prisoners were nothing if not inventive. Stray animals were caught – Harry said stray dogs would enter the cookhouse at their peril. *A large snake, five feet long was killed in the officers' quarters yesterday, and was cleaned and boiled. Those brave enough to eat it said it tasted like chicken!... We have a collection of rather emaciated yaks, two of which are killed off each day, and we have a tasty stew at night.*

Desserts were not forgotten. Fertiliser was used to make a sweet course, apparently full of vitamins. Bananas and pineapples were plentiful and cheap on the island, and they had a regular delivery of pineapples to the mess. *Unfortunately after they have been peeled & the cooks have had their rake-off, there isn't very much left to go on the "pineapple flan".*

They also bought seeds and grew crops. They had flourishing gardens which provided quite a few vegetable and salad items which were vital in supplementing their vitamin-poor diet. Harry managed to find a book about vegetable gardening in Malaya and learned that a local crop, Kane Kong, contains large amounts of vitamin A as well as iron; in addition he found that peanuts are a good source not just of fat and protein, but also vitamins B and C, so that the two together were an excellent combination. However, Harry said that *the leaves which form our veg are almost tasteless and it is like eating grass. The absence of salt is felt, especially in the veg.*

Harry and his friends made the most of any opportunity to acquire food. There are several diary entries which illustrate the importance of food in their lives. *At night shared my bully with Carter's bread. 3 of us had a good tuck-in. Then the padre felt hungry so opened and shared a 'tin of herrings' with him... An RASC officer brought in some yam (turnip) and some mouldy Indian biscuits so there was 'quite a party'... Terrific party full of vitamins – tomato juice, pilchards, salmon, with bread, marg & marmalade-sweetened orange juice & a tin of pineapple each... Had a party at night in Padre's room – herrings, bread, biscuits & jam, & then followed it up with one in mine – bully & rice & marmalade. Felt rather sick.*

These evening 'parties' were social occasions when they talked well into the night discussing the latest rumours about the war and diverse topics including politics, religion and philosophy. Harry frequently said he went to bed feeling full and contented.

Harry also experimented with making interesting brews: *I am making a potent alcoholic drink, ostensibly for its vitamin B content, but raisins, sugar & pineapple juice, if allowed to stand for a few days, make a drink containing more than vit B. These yeast drinks form a very interesting experiment, and consequently more research is required.* He originally concocted it for the Padre's birthday. *"Silman's Special" was the hard drink, & a mighty fine brew it was – I must try it when I get home.* Later in the year he experimented further to make the brew more potent, and he renamed it Panther's Breath.

They occasionally got Red Cross parcels with precious food items including much-prized Marmite, but after the Japanese surrendered at the end of the war, it was found that they had kept a very large proportion of the Red Cross parcels for themselves. Nonetheless, these early entries give the impression that conditions in Changi were reasonably satisfactory for a POW camp. 16th August 1942: *It is now six months since the capitulation – half a year of captivity which on looking back has passed very quickly and not too uncomfortably. Originally, we thought that conditions and food would rapidly deteriorate but on the contrary the food and rations have improved and we can buy almost anything we like from the canteen.*

However, the Japanese never let them forget they were prisoners. *We heard that the C-in-C has been kept in a cell for 4 days without food – no comforts or furniture – & was questioned & re-questioned in the hope that his resistance would break down. The Japs go to both extremes, and one can never be certain whether one will be treated very kindly or biffed over the head with a rifle.*

*

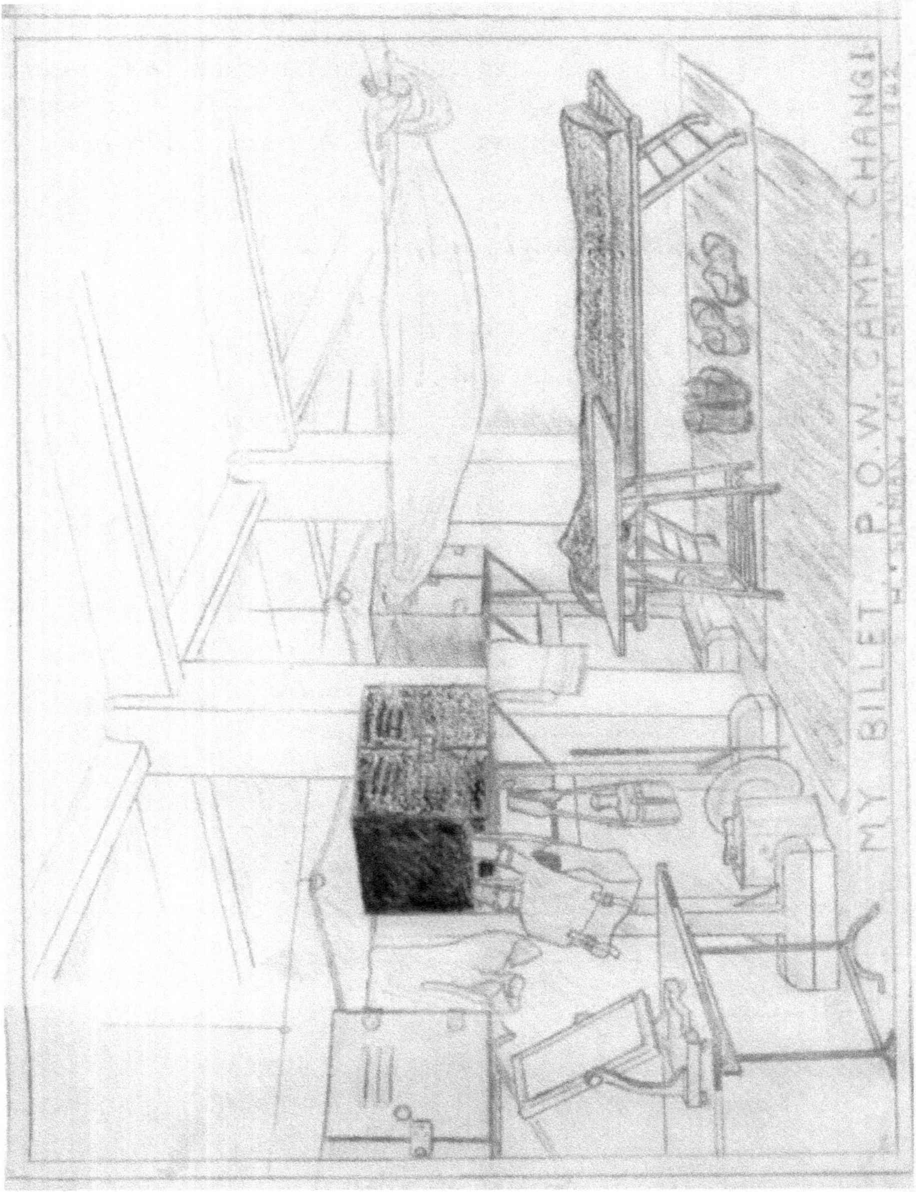
MY BILLET. P.O.W. CAMP. CHANGI.

On Monday afternoon I had the largest sick parade ever...
and was a limp rag when I had finished.

Harry had daily sick parades with large queues of sodden soldiers lining up in the pouring rain, patiently waiting for dressings. Before they began he was given one of the things he missed most – *a really good cup of tea with plenty of milk and sugar in it – not like the watery unsweetened stuff that they put on the table for meal times.*

At these sick parades he saw frequent occurrences of diseases which he had previously only come across in textbooks. He managed to find a tome on tropical diseases which was helpful in adding to the practical knowledge he was gaining on a daily basis. Harry welcomed the opportunity to discuss worrying cases with the other medics in the regular meetings of the Changi Medical Society where the British and Australian doctors shared their findings. Much of their clinical treatment was based on trial and error especially as they were short of the drugs which were needed to effect a cure.

Beriberi, a disease which affected a high proportion of the POWs and caused many deaths, was a major topic for discussion. Harry knew that vitamin B in rice is dissolved out by washing and was their main source of the vitamin in the prison diet. He encouraged the men to eat rice polishings for vitamin B so as to combat beriberi and other vitamin deficiency diseases which were becoming a major problem. Jim Bradley said they found the rice polishings almost unpalatable: 'I think no-one would have attempted to take these, had we not all been so afraid of becoming impotent! The only way to get them down was to put them in a mug, add water, and as they were completely insoluble, swill them down; these rice polishings were nauseating and alive with weevils.'[5] And the medics did not discourage them from eating weevils in the food as they were a source of protein however small!

Harry also suspected that a lack of vitamin B was only part of the picture as some developed beriberi on a good diet while others on a poor diet did not. *The position in regard to vitamins is very serious. About a third of the Battalion is suffering from one form or another of deficiency... I now hear that the so-called Rice Polishings consists of floor sweepings & is not true polishings, containing no B2 and is therefore useless for treatment. If this is the case we are foxed as there are no other remedies to use. The outlook is very grave unless the Japs will provide a good source of B2 for us. One RAOC man developed complete paralysis of his legs in 24 hours – motor & sensory. How little do people in England realise the importance of vitamins in the diet.*

There were other diseases also ascribed to vitamin deficiency such as encephalitis, sprue, pellagra, scrotal dermatitis and stomatitis. Marmite helped to combat some of them but was in woefully short supply. *I called a meeting of the two messing officers & discussed future policy. A memo came out recently stating minimum amounts of peanuts, RP, palm oil & whitebait to be included in the daily diet.* Harry recognised an eye condition caused by vitamin A deficiency. It started off with pain and blurring of vision and if not diagnosed in time, it caused permanent blindness. He also wondered if conjunctivitis which was similarly prevalent might be connected to a vitamin A deficiency.

A real headache for Harry was the number of men with metatarsalgia – acutely painful feet. He was baffled by the fact that they did not show much improvement after a week of large doses of rice polishings, as it was thought the condition was caused by lack of vitamin B. He found it strange that the condition seemed to be more painful when the patients were in bed, and had many discussions with colleagues on the search for a cause and treatment, hoping to do something to relieve the pain and the insomnia it caused.

Another major problem was malaria. The Medical Society gave two lectures a week on malaria which Harry said were very interesting with much new material. *Malaria cases when discharged are now divided into two groups A and B. A are in good condition and would live through another attack, B are in bad condition and may get a deficiency disease and sink after another attack. This latter group will have atebrin twice weekly to ward off attacks.* Harry had recurrent attacks of malaria for several years after he was liberated, probably in common with many ex-POWs.

Harry was upset that there was little he could do in cases which would not have been fatal under normal circumstances. *Scrotal dermatitis caused 2 deaths last week – some cases are very bad and the men roll about in agony on their beds. Marmite seems to help some cases. There is a vast field of research here.*

A dysentery epidemic had started within the first few days of arrival in Changi, and it continued to be a constant cause for concern. A virulent form came in from Singapore and the early poor sanitary conditions and lack of hygiene among the troops contributed to the increase of the infection. It was so common that Harry said it was easy to overlook symptoms of other conditions: *Although not on duty I saw three cases in the evening, including a query appendicitis which I sent to hospital late at night. It is very difficult to distinguish between the abdominal pain of dysentery and a true appendicitis and one must be careful not to miss the latter.*

There was news of an outbreak of cholera in Singapore and Harry said he *took immediate steps to see that all water, vegetables & fruit are boiled. I hope it doesn't spread up to Changi otherwise we are all in a helluva mess. No word of prophylactic inoculation – I doubt whether there is sufficient supply on the island.* The cholera scare was caused by a seaman disembarking in Singapore and the man was quarantined. The authorities took the situation seriously and issued instructions for strict sanitation.

Cholera inoculations were given to the cooks and anyone who handled food, plus all the medical officers. Usually the reaction is slight, but Harry developed a fever after his injection. Vaccine was provided by the Japanese for a second cholera inoculation, although it looked to Harry like a *clear water coloured fluid. As I have had no reaction at all, I suspect it may actually be water.* Harry's misgivings may have been well-founded, as the injections seemed to give little protection less than a year later when they were sent up country.

Cases of diphtheria increased as the incarceration continued, and the hospital wards set aside for these patients soon filled up. It began with the arrival of new POWs who were not isolated. Harry thought it careless that they were allowed to mix and sleep alongside all the other POWs. He said that the fatal nature of diphtheria was apt to be forgotten, and that the MOs who sat on cases of suspected tonsillitis were endangering the lives of men. The shortage of antitoxin and bacteriological facilities were severe drawbacks.

There was a wide variety of work for the medics. One job he did not enjoy was collecting smears for medical examination. *It was my fate last Sat. to be a sticker i.e. for 2 hours I was inserting glass rods into large bottoms pushed into my face, obscuring all other views. The whole proceedings were very unpleasant, and the sight of the colonels and officers with their trousers down was rather humiliating. Everyone took it in good part and joked about it for several days afterwards. I was the butt of numerous jokes!*

Another disagreeable task was *checking the feet & between the toes of the men looking for Singapore foot (not a pleasant pastime esp. after lunch – rather malodorous). Found about 25 new cases – rather a large proportion in our small community – largely due to shower baths & men walking about in bare feet. This is now strictly forbidden.*

Harry's medical notes contained the occasional unusual report: *A fusilier vomited up a roundworm 8" long – he says it gave him a shock! Worms are an oft unsuspected cause of abdominal pain, nausea, vomiting & possibly loss of weight. Worms are quite common in this country.*

At regular periods, prisoners were sent from Changi to Japan. Before they went, the medics had to do thorough inspections, taking blood samples and smears for examination. *The organisation necessary to prepare, number & examine all the specimens is enormous. Besides this, all the luggage will be put through a disinfectant to 60°. Personal kit carried in a pack will be sprayed with carbolic & the person himself will be dipped in disinfectant. They are certainly sparing no effort to make sure that we take no disease into Japan.* An amusing sight was to see the small Japanese MO having to stand on tiptoe to prick the ears of the tall British Tommies for the blood sample they wanted.

Not surprisingly, the medical officers themselves were not immune from illness. Harry had a severe attack of dengue, a tropical disease spread by mosquitoes, and was ill for ten days. When he started to feel like eating again, some well-meaning friends brought him a half-tin of sardines, opened the previous day, which unfortunately led to severe gastro-enteritis for Harry and two of his companions. They became severely dehydrated and were sent in an ambulance to hospital. *There was much consternation amongst the officers and spectators who saw us being taken away as we looked almost moribund. After a wait of ¾ hour in the reception office, we were carried up 3 flights of stairs by four non-co-operative stretcher bearers & my life was in danger of being suddenly ended. Fortunately the attack soon settled down.*

*

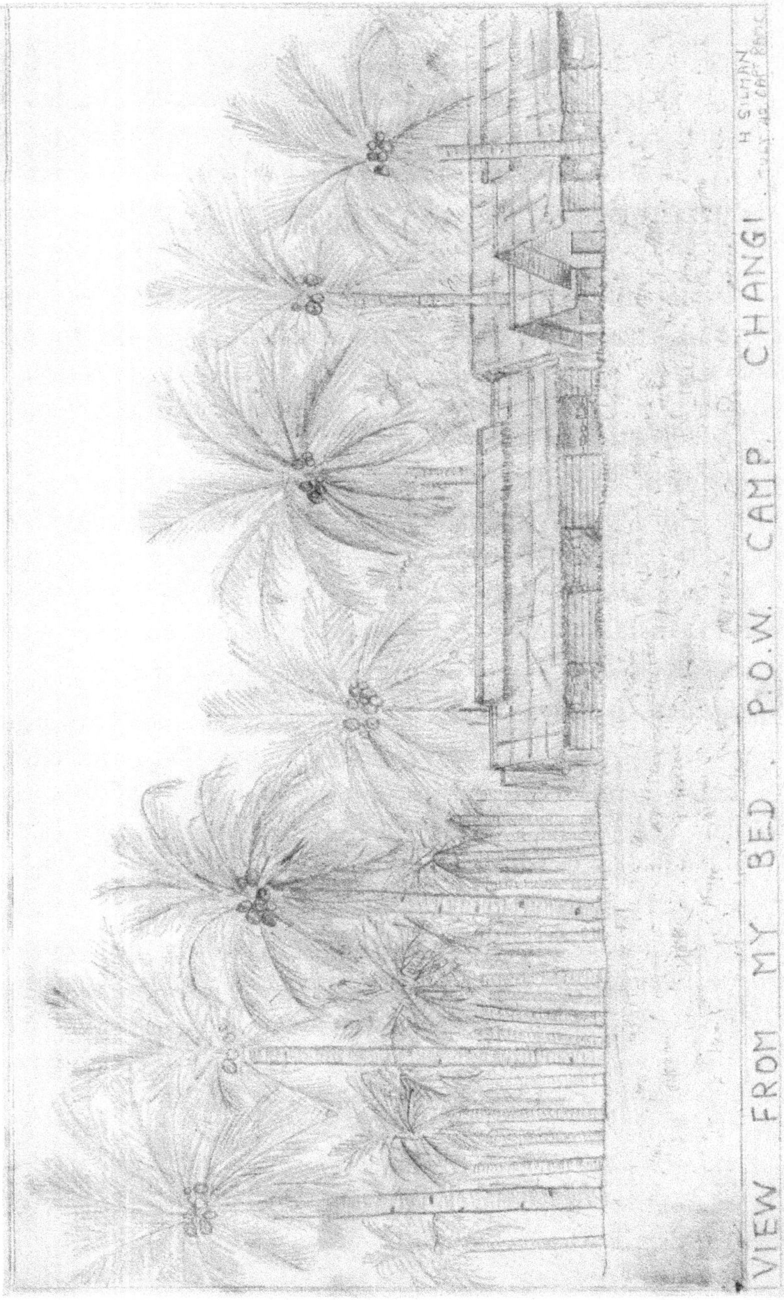
VIEW FROM MY BED. P.O.W. CAMP. CHANGI
H SILMAN

It is strange how men have turned to religion
for mental comfort while a POW

The Japanese were quite happy for the POWs to follow their religious customs. Indeed, they actively encouraged it, perhaps because they respected religion, perhaps because it kept the prisoners occupied. In any event, even when other privileges were withdrawn, religious services were not affected.

Harry was very friendly with the Padre. They were both attached to the regiment as against being regular soldiers, and they were both fully occupied in their respective positions. Each appreciated the other's role. Through the internet, I was able to contact Padre's daughter Louise Reynolds, and learnt that her father equally valued his friendship with Harry. Louise sent me a copy of her father's diary and her research into his memoirs gave me an insight into his work.

Within 24 hours of being taken prisoner, Padre Eric Cordingly found a little mosque, once used for Indian troops who used to live in the area, and knew that it would be well suited as a church as it was light and cool. By the end of the week, skilled volunteers had lovingly made a pulpit and altar, and produced seating and furnishings. They designed tin tubes to look like candles that held small tin cups for an oil/paraffin mix. When lit, he said they were hardly distinguishable from real candles. Later a beautiful brass cross was fashioned from a howitzer shell case, and this cross was taken from camp to camp as the prisoners were moved. When the war ended Padre took the cross back home to the UK, but in 1992 the family returned it to Changi museum.

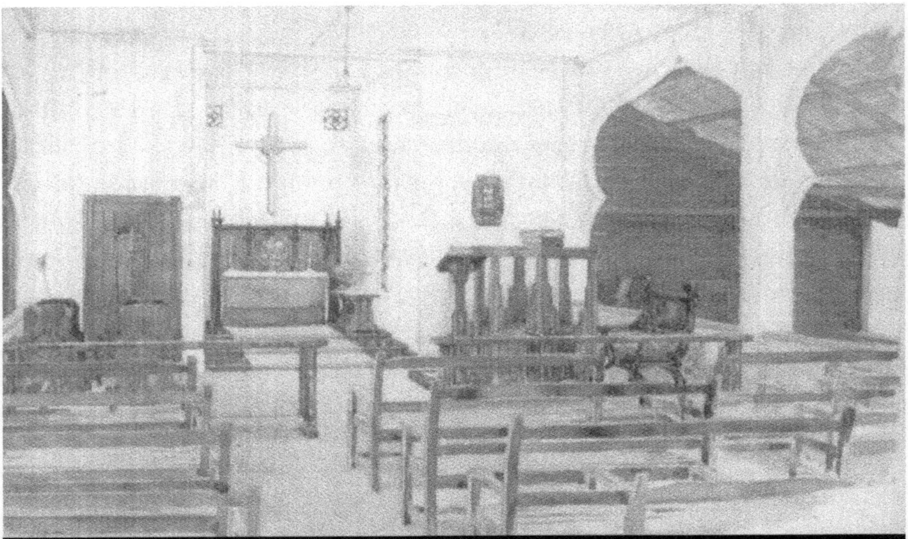

Interior of Padre Cordingly's St George's Chapel in converted mosque (E. Stacy)

Padre's Sunday services were very well attended, as were various discussion groups during the week which finished with a simple service at the end of each day. Easter and Christmas services were especially meaningful. Eric Cordingly said for him, it was 'a wonderful time in my life in spite of the grim times'. A large proportion of the men appreciated the spiritual consolation offered by the regular services, and he wrote in his diary that he never felt more needed. He kept an accurate account of all the funerals he had organised, and after he was repatriated, he spent many months writing to the families of the prisoners he had cared for before they died.

Harry was from an orthodox Jewish family, and although not overly observant, he quickly identified a need to have weekly Shabbat (Sabbath) services and keep, as far as possible, the age-old traditions of the festivals. It is interesting that although in Japanese eyes all prisoners were the lowest of the low, there was virtually no incidence of anti-Semitism. There was some concern when a nominal roll of all Jewish personnel was requested, as many men thought it might lead to a similar situation as in Europe, but it was purely for record purposes. Harry learned that the percentage of Jews in the army was 0.5%, which was higher than he thought and he was able to find people in different areas who would take responsibility for Jewish burial services if necessary.

Harry was somewhat surprised to find that he became the spokesman for the Jewish prisoners as the majority were non-practising. He organised the first of what would be regular Friday night services in Changi. To start with, these were held wherever they could find a suitable place: *Attended my first army religious service – strange that it should be as a prisoner of war. I was the only officer, 1 Sergeant, 1 Corporal and about 16 ORs. No-one had a prayer book so we had a short stand up service – three men each reciting a bit of a prayer that they could remember. The service was held at 8pm in a rubber plantation behind some distant billets. We couldn't sit down owing to the ants.*

As they had no prayer books, Harry arranged for the men to write out the prayers they could remember for the following week, and hoped they could have a more satisfactory service. This was held in a small sports pavilion out in the woods. *It started in a typical fashion 30 minutes late – one man had a siddur* (prayer book) *and acted as chazan* (cantor who leads the congregation) *so that we had a fairly good service. Two men with good voices acted as the nucleus of a choir and led the singing. After such absence from services it will take a little while before the words become familiar again.*

It took a couple of weeks before they could find a more suitable venue for their service. Harry was greatly relieved when the senior Padre called in on him in the MI room and offered his little church near Division HQ for the Friday night services, *a very decent gesture*.

Attendance improved greatly at the weekly services, although Harry was disappointed that only a few of the Jewish officers turned up.

It is strange how men have turned to religion for mental comfort while a POW. The Padre has services morning & night, & crowded services on Sunday. It gives a certain feeling of relief & satisfaction to lift up one's voice in hymns etc. It is a pity we haven't sufficient prayer books & a good chazan so that we could do that.

David Arkush, a dentist, was from an orthodox Jewish family and his father was a chazan. He joined the small congregation soon after the start. He had brought his prayer book with him and made a highly valued contribution to the services before he was sent away. *Capt Arkush of ADC gave them a short talk afterwards about Jewish life in Singapore. He hopes to give them similar talks after each service. It is a good idea and helps them to remember their faith and upbringing.*

The first day of Rosh Hashanah (the Jewish New Year) had a record attendance. Harry said that *owing to the limitations imposed by the prayer book it is difficult to give a true service but we managed to put bits and pieces together and all in all, it worked out very well.*

Ten days later was Yom Kippur, the Day of Atonement and normally a fast day. Harry thought there would not be many who would fast this year and he himself would not encourage it under the prison camp circumstances, leaving it to each man's choice. This High Holy Day service meant a lot to him: *yesterday was the most remarkable Yom Kippur I have ever spent. We had two services, a long morning one and a shorter afternoon one. There were over 70 present in the morning including a few RAF newly arrived. Capt. Phillips had prepared an anglicised service. We read a portion about Isaac in English. There were about 10 officers present – many of whom I had never seen before. One of the men asked us if we could finish by 12.30 as they had to back for 1 o'clock for dinner! A few observed the day strictly, but those that didn't can be forgiven for it was terrifically hot & sweat was pouring out of us as we stood listening.*

Over the years in Changi, services were held in a variety of venues including the Sergeants' Mess and a cinema in the hospital grounds.

In January 1943 a Dutch rabbi, Rabbi Chaim Nussbaum, from Indonesia came into the camp. He conducted services and kept a record of the festivals which were celebrated as best they could, sometimes with a considerable amount of ingenuity. *2 nights ago I attended a Seder service* (special prayers and meal for the festival of Pesach/Passover) *– a remarkably successful affair. Nussbaum is a genius for overcoming difficulties. We had matzo made out of sago flour, wine made from fermented rice water. The four cups consisted of coffee owing to the shortage of wine. Charoseth was grated coconut and sugar, maror was mint leaves, and for hard-boiled eggs we had spinach leaves. Somehow Pesach doesn't seem the same without hard-boiled eggs. However it all made me feel quite homesick and over coffee and smokes at the end, we sang the usual songs and broke up after a very merry evening.* Rabbi Nussbaum gave Harry a siddur which he treasured greatly and brought back from the war.

Whenever Harry wrote about the festivals, it is clear his thoughts turned to home. *As I walked to the service I thought of everyone at home and felt sure that they would at the same time be thinking about me and under what circumstances I was living. It is at times like this that one thinks of one's family & vice versa.*

*

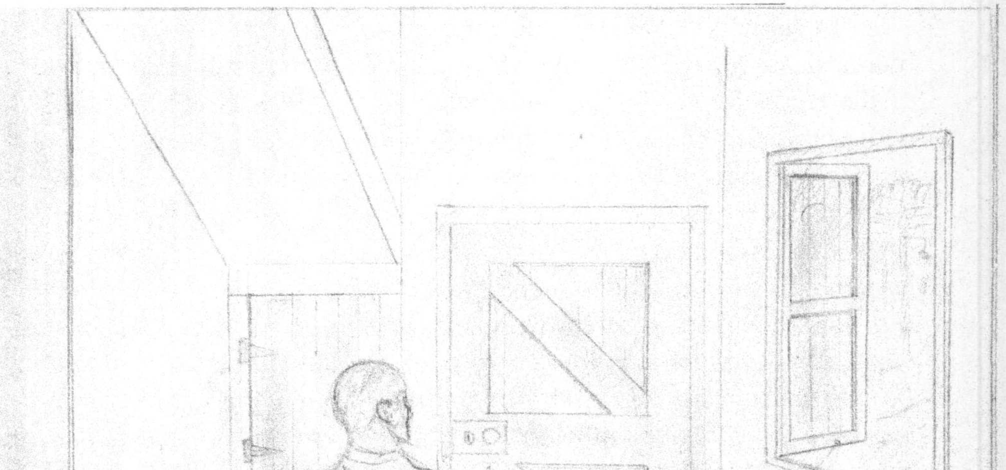
COMBINED STUDY AND CANTEEN CHANGI P.o.W.C.

Idleness is a curse and is one of the worst features of the POW camp.

Harry felt he was lucky being a Medical Officer as it filled a large part of his day. *Most of my time is occupied. The other officers and men find that time hangs heavily on their hands... Idleness is a curse and is one of the worst features of the POW camp. It gives men too much time to sit and think and brood. I am only too glad to get into a chair or bed to rest after a long session in the MI Room.*

Maintaining the morale of the prisoners in Changi was considerably helped by the frequent concert parties. With such a huge prison population there was a wealth of talent, not only in musicians, actors, singers and variety acts, but also with people who had backstage skills in lighting, sound and set design. One of the captives was Ronald Searle. Although most famous for his cartoons and caricatures – after the war he published a graphic pictorial account of the horrors endured by POWs in the Far East – he was responsible for the programme design and professional scenery for many of the shows.

Harry enjoyed every production he saw. These included Dover Road, The Dancing Years and Badgers Green, a play about village life that had been successful in London. He was held spellbound by the dramatic last scene in The Monkey's Paw, and he rated each show very highly commenting on the excellent scenery and costumes. After the opening night of I Killed the Count, he wrote: *the scenery and decor could not have been better even in a London show. The Sappers made the scenery and converted old furniture into modern stuff. The acting was of a very high standard. The star performer as the Chief Inspector had a very long part to learn and was word perfect. They have been unfortunately stricken with illness and each day some member of the cast gets ill and they have to rehearse it all over again with the new addition. This must be very tiring.*

Harry, with friends from the 18th Division, went over to a different section to see Shaw's play Arms & the Man. *It was an open air show in a grassy hollow with scenery made out of twigs & leaves – very ingeniously constructed portions fixed into slots in the ground. The actors had a remarkable variety of makeshift uniforms & dresses. Although the play was written 40 years ago, many passages were strangely topical & could have been applied to the Jap-British fight. Five minutes before the end it started to pour down, so that the play ended prematurely & in some disorder.*

Each group was allocated a specific day to see the Division concert, and Harry's group had to accept untimely endings quite frequently because of the weather. One of these shows was aptly named Rain or Shine.

On another occasion he had a seat in the front row. *The compere, with a serious face, announced during the show "Is there a doctor in the house?" I knew the old joke but as I was pointed out he asked me the introit "How do you like the show Doc?" There was a tremendous burst of laughter and cheering, and now everywhere I go I am greeted with that phrase. The compere told some of the dirtiest jokes I have ever heard in my life. The men enjoyed them but the colonels were very annoyed.*

Some of the performers went on to become well-known in show business after they were released. Sydney Piddington was a thought-reader who entertained the troops. After the war he and his wife performed as the Piddingtons, and were world-famous for their

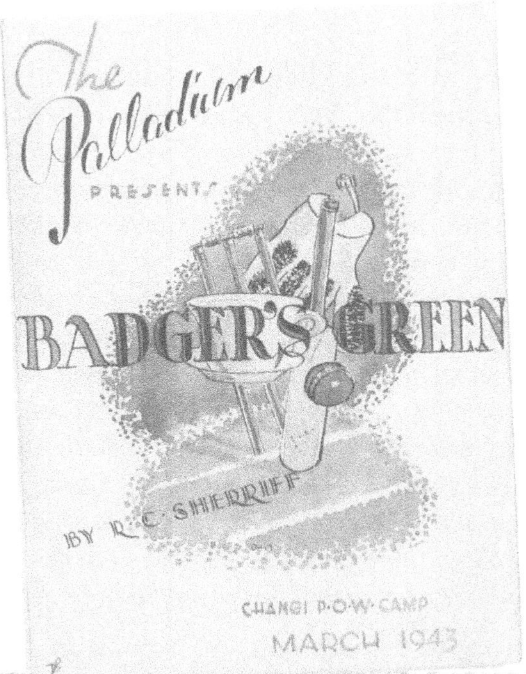
The Palladium
PRESENTS
BADGER'S GREEN
BY R. C. SHERRIFF
CHANGI P.O.W. CAMP
MARCH 1943

BADGERS GREEN.

by
R.C.SHERIFF.

CAST.
In order of appearance.

Doctor Wetherby..........Capt.T.M.Mitchell.
Maid........................Lieut.D.Barbour.
Mr.Twigg.................Lieut.J.L.Mackwood.
Major Forrester..........Capt.C.P.Wilkinson.
Dickie Wetherby..........Capt.J.C.Atcherly.
Mr.Butler....................Major W.W.Auld.
Mr.Butler's Secretary.......Lieut.R.M.Adie.
Rogers - The Landlord.....MajorJ.M.Spears.
Gardener........................Pte.R.White.
Mrs.Wetherby........Capt.R.Fitz-Barrington.
Mrs.Evans....................Gnr.D.R.Cooper.
George.......................Lieut.D.H.Higgs.
Charlie......................Lieut.F.J.White.

o-o-o-o-o-o-o-o

The Play produced by F.W.Bradshaw.

o-o-o-o-o-o-o-o

For the
Eighteenth Divisional Players.

Stage Manager - Chris Buckingham.
Scenic Artist - Ronald Searle.
Electrician - Ben Foster.
Carpenter - Harry Craig.

o-o-o-o-o-o-o-o

SYNOPSIS OF THE SCENES.

Act 1, Scene 1, The Library of Dr.Wetherby's House at Badgers Green.

Act 2, Scene 1, The Same - following day.

Act 2 Scene 2, The same - a little later.

Act 3, Scene 1, Inside the Marquee at the Cricket Match on the Village Green, on the morning of the Match.

Act 3, Scene 2, The Same, during and after the Cricket Match.

o-o-o-o-o-o-o-o

For the
Palladium Theatre.

House Manager - Alan R.Bush.

Box Office Manager - Jack Milnes Wood.

o-o-o-o-o-o-o-o

Badgers Green programme showing Ronald Searle as the Scenic Artist telepathy act. Harry went to a couple of thought-reading acts but was very sceptical. *Last night the Dutch thought-reader made a return visit. I bet the Padre 20 cigs beforehand that it was all a fake & was done by using an accomplice in the room. I decided on a test & gave sealed instructions to Doc Emery who was acting as the medium, so that only Emery & myself knew what he had to do. After a lot of fumbling, he performed the task written down. This completely shattered my disbelief & scepticism. With my scientific education, I have hitherto refused to believe anything supernatural, anything that could not be explained by ordinary laws of physics, chemistry, etc. The existence of God came into the argument with the Padre, who argued that just because he couldn't prove scientifically the presence of a God, it doesn't mean to say that there isn't one. The experiment last night shows that there are still lots of phenomena that cannot be explained in our present state of knowledge & there may be something in spiritualism etc.*

He also attended a demonstration of hypnotism. *A young medical orderly was hypnotised after only 30 seconds and was kept under for 30 minutes. He was as stiff as a log and was suspended between two chairs, and a heavy man jumped on his middle without bending him. I examined the boy while he was under the influence and was much impressed. He was in a state of tonic contraction, (except his arms which were flaccid), his pupils were fixed and dilated – insensitive to pain – P and R normal. He came round quite easily and except for feeling very tired there were no after effects. He described a sensation as of electric shocks going through him and he was helpless and unable to move. He then remembered nothing till he woke up. This demonstration of Hypnotism and the previous one of Thought-Reading, both by Dutchmen, have made me a believer in the occult. I am now willing to believe anything!*

Perhaps the most popular performers were the female impersonators. Gloria D'Earie had been a well-known drag act before

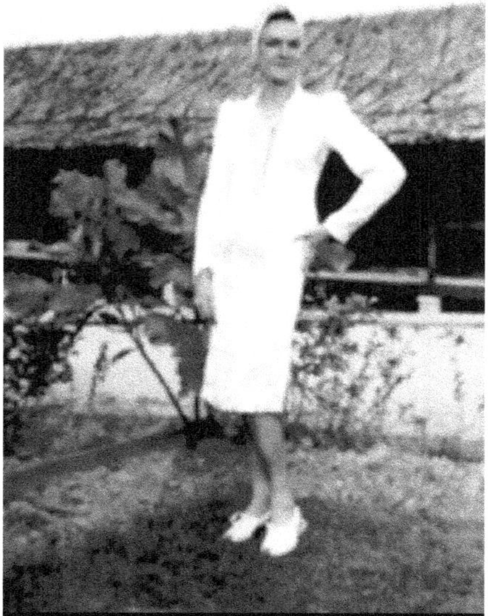
Gloria D'Earie

the war. When Harry saw her he said *she was more feminine than a girl. The Apache dance was a perfect one & "she" was always graceful & light. She talked, sang & danced like a girl.* There were several entertainers who were very willing to dress as women including a successful Australian performer who was known as 'Judy' (Garland). They managed to obtain make-up left behind by nurses when they evacuated the island, and when this ran out, the chemists were able to manufacture substitutes. Some shows would end with the 'lady' lifting up his skirt to reveal his male credentials. Apparently, some of the female impersonators were so successful, the Japanese guards would dash backstage to check for themselves that no women had been smuggled into the camp.

The performers were careful to omit specific sections overtly critical of the Japanese if they saw they were attending the concerts. As a general rule, the material in the shows was not censored in advance, apart from banning the singing of the National Anthem which the Japanese thought would encourage demonstrations of patriotism. So instead, the producers of the shows substituted Land of Hope and Glory.

Sport flourished in Changi. There were several elite sportsmen among the prisoners who hoped to revive their careers at the end of the war, and they organised soccer, rugby, hockey, cricket, baseball and basketball matches. Watching the American seamen playing baseball,

Harry said that hearing the US twang and expressions was just like a scene in a film. There was always some game to watch. *The officers played the NCO at football – the former seemed to spend most of their time on the ground. Some of them had sticking plaster on various parts of their anatomies in the evening.*

There was a degree of rivalry between the Australian and British POWs and Harry enjoyed watching an Aussies v. British cricket match in spite of the fact *that they scored over 200 for 4 declared and we were all out for 60. It was amazing to see in a POW camp, spectators sitting around in long cane chairs, some with sunshades, and watching 'test cricket'.*

Harry was mainly an observer rather than participant in sporting events. However he took golf lessons from a fellow POW who was an assistant pro before the war. Harry said *I can now hit a reasonable straight drive. How long I can do this is a matter of speculation.* The golf instruction came in useful as Harry was a keen golfer well into his 70s.

To begin with they were allowed to go swimming on Changi beach. It involved climbing over barbed wire and negotiating patches of oil, but it was a welcome respite from the monotony of camp life. The Japanese stopped this for a time, but later reinstated the privilege. *First bathing party for many months. It was a long walk about 2 miles – not very pleasant water, rather dirty & barbed wire on concealed bottom step made it a dangerous business. I cut my knees & legs in a few places. Still it was a good change & I got a little exercise out of it.*

The prisoners were quite ingenious in making the best of the materials to hand. In one of the early days, Harry spent the afternoon making himself a pair of slippers from an old tyre which was an arduous task as he had to cut through the thick rubber. Three days later he started to make himself a cap from a pair of battledress trousers. This was also hard work and took him a few days. When he wore it for the first time, he was relieved there were no caustic comments.

At one point Harry decided to try to grow a moustache. He said he had thoughts of Errol Flynn as he cultivated it. However *as day succeeded day, it looked more like a rat-bitten toothbrush so this morning it came off mid much wailing and moaning.*

Most afternoons Harry was free from medical duties, so he would change into his blue shorts and home-made slippers and potter about doing odd jobs, till about 6 o'clock when he had a shower in time for dinner. He had no problem filling his time. *I have started drawing in fine perspective style my portion of the billet – it will always be engraved on my mind, but the drawing will help.* He said there was general appraisal when he completed this, his first drawing since he left school, and it *exceeded my most sanguine expectations.*

Harry had a number of diary entries detailing his vain efforts at finding the definitive fly paper which would solve the perennial fly problem. *In pm carried on with my fly-paper experiments – very enjoyable as it involves cutting up (and eating) coconuts... Most of my furniture is very sticky following my experiments on fly catching fluids. Am using various combinations of castor oil, coconut oil, cachou nut resin and the scummy stuff from the Jack-fruit tree. No success so far.*

A popular institution was what was known as the 'Changi University'. Officers gave lectures on their specialist subjects and there was a huge variety on offer including Economics, Law, Maths, Theology and several languages. *The lectures are now in full swing & the whole place has a studious atmosphere with the fellows walking about with books & pads under their arms. Even the General is attending the theology lectures.*

Harry chose to study German, mainly because it did not clash with his sick parades. He took it seriously, practising sometimes for four to five hours in his spare time. Books in modern languages were scarce, so he borrowed a German grammar book and copied it out in full. Even before the university classes started, he had been studying from a teach-yourself German book. He was introduced to a young Swiss man by the Padre, and arranged to spend an hour each day with him for conversation. He felt he had mastered sufficient knowledge to keep German conversation going, and clearly had achieved quite a reasonable standard as he was able to read a couple of books in German with the aid of a dictionary.

Harry also studied Italian and was pleased he could converse with his Italian patients who, he wrote, came to him with the most obscure complaints. It is clear Harry enjoyed studying languages as he talked about learning Russian from native speakers in the camp, and basic Japanese from a self-teaching handbook. He kept up with his schoolboy French by reading some simple French books which were available.

The POWs had pooled their books to form an eclectic library and Harry spent much spare time reading a wide variety of fiction and non-fiction. These included medical tomes, Churchill's speeches in Hansard, and novels by many authors including A A Milne, P G Wodehouse, Marguerite Steen and Sapper's Bulldog Drummond books. He read Haldane's Science in Wartime but was not happy with *the way he mixes science & Socialism. Everything that's new, good or progressive he attributes to Lenin, Marx & USSR, and anything vaguely bad or wrong he blames Tories, Chamberlain or Capitalists. It is remarkable for a man to use politics as examples in a scientific book.*

During the first few weeks in Changi, he found it quite hard concentrating for long periods on a book, and said that other people had the same difficulty. However as he adjusted to prison life, he wrote *I am improving the shining hour by delving deep into the library –*

mainly English literature, geography & history. I am rather pleased with myself that I can now sit down & enjoy a book that I formerly would have called "heavy".

There was a series of lectures on general subjects given at Changi Cinema. Harry attended a lecture on earthquakes. *Most hopeful part is that Japan has a big quake about once every 20 years – her time is now up.* There were also lectures on car maintenance which Harry thought would be useful after the war, although he said one motor lecture was given by *a dopey lecturer who seemed to fall asleep in the middle of sentences & was constantly dropping things out of his hand – must be pathological.*

One talk he really enjoyed was given by the Australian wicket-keeper Barnett on his Test match experiences. *He spoke for quite a while about that exciting Test match at Leeds, when they won on the 3rd day and I knelt on the gravel all day watching them. He had a fund of good stories to relate.*

He particularly relished the lectures on current affairs, and noted in detail the topics discussed. Combined with the news gleaned from the illegal radios, Harry had a good knowledge of the battles in Europe and North Africa. One lecture was given by General Percival on the BEF in France and the reasons for their failure. After learning from another talk about the disastrous battle of Mersa Matruh in Egypt which the army barely survived, he commented that *it came as a shock to us – each defeat & each evacuation increases the duration of our stay here. It is a remarkable thing when one comes to recount British victories on land in this war. How we always muddle through to victory is amazing.*

Harry and his friends would chat about the lectures and latest news. *It is very pleasant to sit out in the cool of the evening on the verandah or on the grass in front of the billet. We discuss the cause of our failures, individual deeds of bravery and otherwise; our future, and rumours which are numerous and often far-fetched. Some most remarkable rumours spread round and are believed by many of the troops eg The Russians are fighting on German soil, there has been an invasion of England, etc. It is impossible to trace the source of these "authentic" rumours.*

Many of their moonlight discussions after the 'nocturnal feed' were related to war. *Padre is firstly of the impression that war is not inevitable & will soon cease to exist as men become more civilised. I argued that history always repeats itself – there will always be wars & that in some countries, civilisation is going backward. The nature of man cannot be altered & the bad side occasionally comes to the top with will to power → war.*

Sometimes their choice of topic for discussion seemed to be quite random. *Argued until early hours of morning why water climbs up a capillary tube. Tried to remember my physics – problem remained unsolved.*

Harry played bridge regularly, and gave a series of bridge lessons to would-be players. He started a bridge competition which was popular. Some Dutch officers who were billeted in the same building were regular opponents. *I have played bridge several times against 2 very good Dutch players – their Smith 4NT convention baffles me & also them at times.* Bridge was played in the evenings which had its disadvantages: *Played bridge on verandah as usual but extended the hours of play till 10pm by using my hurricane lamp. Drawback is the large number of little insects and animals that collect around the light.*

Every evening would have some arranged activity. *We are a cheerful little crowd & have pleasant sessions in the evening.* When there were blackouts, they entertained themselves playing word games and quizzes.

Harry's 32nd birthday and his first as a POW was celebrated in style on 21st December 1942. He received a number of gifts and as lavish a supper party for his friends as they could manage. He had an expensive cake made by the officers' mess cookhouse, but unfortunately *it collapsed in the morning & had to be supported with string & bumph – tastefully cut to make it appear decorative.* There was enough of Harry's *very tasty & alcoholic Panther's Breath brew for everyone. All*

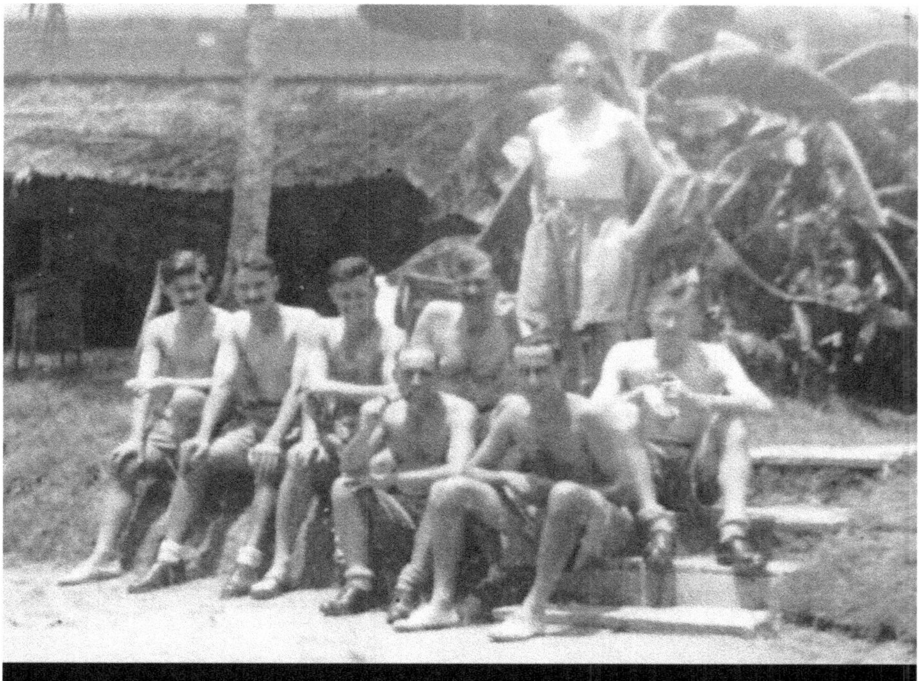

Group photo: Harry second from right (sitting)

in all it was a good night's work & my first birthday in a POW camp. I wonder how many more there will be. None I hope!

It is understandable that the prisoners of war made the most of every opportunity for a celebration, but none more so than Christmas, a joint celebration by the British and the Dutch. On Christmas Eve, on the green in front of the mess, there was a grand sacred concert organised by the Dutch. *It looked like a crowded fairground from our position on the balcony. It ended up with the fire ceremony, which is a symbolic affair – the fire represents the spirit of life and freedom which keeps burning, and the Dutch 'broadcast' a message to their wives and families in front of the fire, and then each one took a burning rod and lit a candle in his own tent. The association of flame with life is a very common one in many religions. It was quite a dramatic affair, as all the lights were doused, and only the flickering fire played on the announcer's face.*

Harry described this first Christmas Day in captivity as *a day of mutual compliments and bright atmosphere. There is a tremendous menu arranged which will satisfy every gourmand and gourmet.* One of the highlights of their Christmas dinner was the absence of rice! It consisted of *chicken soup, fish creole, roast chicken, and 3 veg including new potatoes, Xmas pudding, savoury, wine (home-made).* The cooks had obviously been planning this festive meal for some time.

At midday the British entertained the Dutch officers to coffee and cakes, and after dinner, about 25 British officers joined the Dutch for another party. *Mutual congratulation speeches were made by the respective OCs, and we stood in silence for various reasons on numerous occasions eg Dutch royal family, Dutch wives, allied casualties, etc. Harris made a very optimistic speech in which he said that by June '43 we would be victorious, and that next Xmas we would be out of here. Time will tell.*

Christmas inevitably turned everyone's thoughts to home. *There were many sad faces today as they read the various messages issued by various commanders. They all have one thing in common, hoping that by next Xmas we will be by our own fireside.*

New Year's Eve was another justification for a party. This was held in Padre's room. *We finished off the meal by a toast to the New Year, drunk with a mixture of the Jap 'brandy', Padre's communion wine and pineapple juice. The Jap stuff was almost raw spirit, and we got about ½ cupful each. It made the troops very hilarious, and at midnight we went out and shook hands with all and sundry. There were the usual songs e.g. Auld Lang Syne, followed by Blaydon Races, We're Here Because We're Here, etc. Led by a bloke banging on a tin box, the men marched up and down outside till nearly 2 am singing and carousing. The Dutch downstairs also entered into the spirit of the thing, and altogether we passed from the old into the new year in traditional style.*

Chapter Six

Selarang

We have taken part in an incident
unparalleled in Military History.

For the first six months of captivity, POW life continued fairly uneventfully. There were frequent instances of mean-spirited bullying and temporary restrictions of liberties, with a few isolated incidents of torture. Typical of the guards' unreasonable behaviour was this scene: *Hedley, trying to be helpful in his capacity as amateur interpreter, put his foot in it with a Jap Corporal who proceeded to give Adrian a hell of a bashing with his fist, feet and rifle. This went on for several minutes and a large crowd of onlookers gathered round. It is very humiliating mentally besides the physical damage and Adrian behaved splendidly and bore it all with very good grace.* However the prisoners learnt strategies they hoped would avoid upsetting the guards and they coped with what were mainly petty punishments.

The number of POWs in Changi had also dropped substantially as large groups were regularly shipped off to forced labour in Japan and the Dutch East Indies (now Indonesia), and also to work on the Burma Railway. It was rare there was any news of these men, although there was much speculation about their fate. Occasionally survivors from places such as Java turned up in Changi, with dreadful tales to tell of vicious treatment by the Japanese, but in general life in the camp was fairly stable. This continued until what history books have recorded as the Selarang Incident.

On September 6th 1942 Harry wrote that they had taken part *in an incident unparalleled in military history.* Four prisoners had attempted an escape from Changi but had been recaptured. Japan had not ratified the Geneva Convention which specified standards for the humanitarian treatment of prisoners of war. These included acceptable punishment after an escape attempt. In fact it was widely considered that prisoners of war had a moral duty to try to escape, and those caught should be liable to disciplinary punishment only.

After the abortive escape, the Japanese insisted that all the Changi POWs should sign a 'parole' agreeing not to escape. This would contravene one of the terms of the Geneva Convention, so they all refused to sign, and as punishment the whole POW camp was sent to Selarang barracks. Although this number did not include the 2,500 sick and dying in the camp hospital, many more were unfit and had enormous difficulties on the two-mile march to Selarang.

Not knowing whether we would come back or not, all stores as far as possible were taken, reserve rations were given out, library books and tools were scattered among the men, medical stores were loaded on the ambulance which also towed two full water tank trucks – loaded full, with kit, sick men, tables etc.

The motley procession that set off was a remarkable sight. Ovens, stoves, containers were all taken including firewood and rations on small trucks loaded to a height of 10-12 feet. Men carried their belongings slung on bamboo poles and the move was carried out in good spirit, the men being very cheerful and light-hearted. The C-in-C complimented the men on this in an Order of the Day. We didn't know what to do with our livestock so the ducks were carried upside down by officers and the chickens were left.

It is fortunate they took so much with them as their provisions helped to supplement the meagre rations they were given. Selarang barracks had originally been built to accommodate 1,600 men. Now it was to hold 17,000. The Japanese restricted the area even further, excluding all the existing latrines. This meant that there was an immediate necessity to dig fresh latrines through the concrete square into which they were all crammed.

Harry described the first night there: *Flies were increasing in number and swill etc was accumulating. Latrines were dug through concrete all through the first night; the men worked like Trojans, digging long rows of trenches 16ft deep while the sappers made latrine tops from doors of billets, men were sleeping on the roofs and all over the courtyard except for space for cookhouses and latrines. The road running round the billet was out of bounds and the Jap sentries beat up anyone treading on the road. A machine gun was mounted on one corner and surrounded with barbed wire. There was no protection from the rain.*

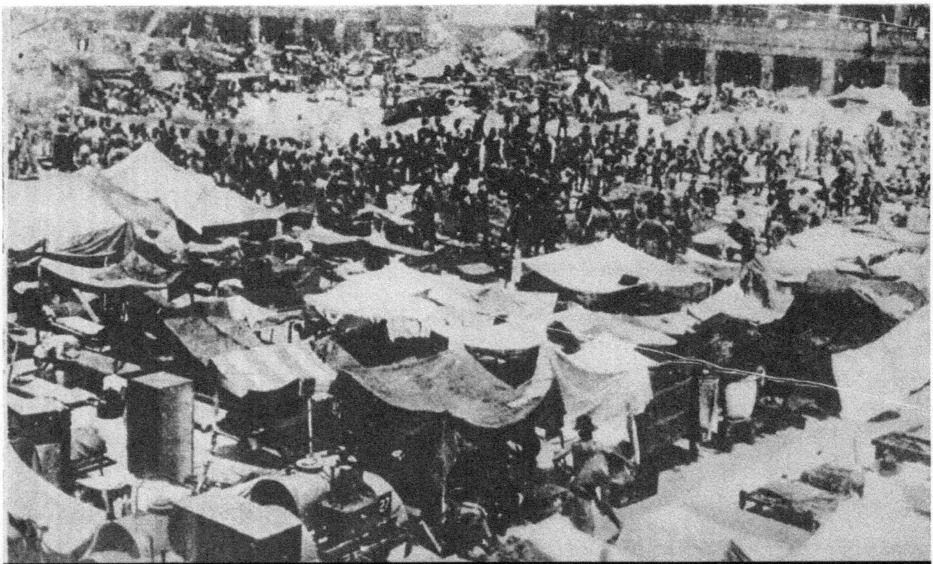

Selarang barracks

The Japanese promised 'measures of severity': two water taps and one concrete well supplied water for all 17,000, and they had to queue for up to four hours to get the day's strict ration. There was an order forbidding the use of water for washing or shaving, and it was clear there would be further outbreaks of dysentery. Each man had a sleeping space of 6ft by 2ft. Thousands slept outside on the concrete with no protection from the rain.

Despite all the deprivation, Harry described the wonderful spirit of the men. *It was an amazing sight. The courtyard looked like Hyde Park with its flickering lights, concerts going on in every corner, pianos playing for sing-songs, men feverishly digging latrines by lamp light.* Jim Bradley[5] said the guards could not understand how they could put on a concert show and said that 'the pluck of these men in such appalling conditions was totally incomprehensible to them'.

There was no suitable MI room so Harry took his meagre stores to the ambulance van and rigged up a little medical room there. He could only see urgent and acute cases, and no ordinary dressings or treatments were done. The Australians had set up a hospital tent in the middle of the courtyard, and were doing dentistry and operations. An acute appendectomy was done the first night by lamplight as the Japanese said 'no communication with hospital'.

The next day food rations were cut to a third but there was still deadlock. Then senior officers were forced to witness the brutal killing of the four escapees. Harry describes this atrocity: *The worst feature of the day was the shooting of the four men who tried to escape. Two Aussies, one RAOC and one Gordon Highlander (two of them were in hospital with malaria and were dragged out of bed) were taken to the seashore and kept waiting for 30 minutes in the boiling sun. A firing party consisted of 4 Sikhs. The Division Commanders and the ACG were summoned to watch. The ACG was allowed a few minutes with each man first. He said that their bearing was wonderful, stood up straight, refused bandages to the eyes and although wounded in the arms and legs by the first few shots remained standing till mortally wounded. It took about 20 minutes and 27 shots were fired – a beastly and brutal affair. The Sikhs then had to bury the dead. This demonstration was supposed to cower us.*

The Japanese said rations would be cut by a third, water by a half and the accommodation by a third until they gave in. *The important question was a medical one, whether we could keep on living under such circumstances. All the latrine space was bound to be used up fairly soon and men were already making a mess over most of the area. Without proper washing facilities, diseases spread by direct contact as well as by flies were a grave danger. There were diphtheria contacts scattered among the men and there was no antitoxin for treatment… The medical authorities estimated that after a month there would be up to 50% dead from dysentery and the remainder would probably be too weak to carry on the essential fatigues, eg fetching water, cooking, cleaning, making latrines etc. It was obvious to any sane man that we couldn't hold out very long under those conditions and reluctantly the C-in-C agreed to sign under duress.*

As the parole had been signed under duress, it was not valid in Allied eyes, but the POWs were allowed to return to Changi. Harry wrote *settled down to normal, brushed out the dust, unpacked and had a shower and a clean change of clothing and everything was again as before. The organ and prayer desk were safely brought back by the Padre and his willing band of helpers. The only ones to be put out by our return were the birds who appeared to have inhabited our billet during our absence. However we are now back safe and sound and it is a closed chapter.*

The Japanese General Fukuei who had ordered the unlawful, inhumane killing of the escapees was himself executed for war crimes on exactly the same spot in April 1946.

The Selarang Incident is said to be the closest concentration of human beings since the Black Hole of Calcutta.

Chapter Seven

Up Country

Hell in the Jungle

For many years, companies from different countries had tried to build a railway from Singapore through Malaya, Thailand and Burma into India. All the plans had failed because of the difficult terrain of dense jungle and high mountains. With the Japanese success in war, there were thousands of POWs who were an excellent source of unpaid labour which, again, was contrary to the Geneva Convention which forbids using POWs for forced labour.

Japan needed the railway to bring their soldiers and supplies up to the Burma-India border. They estimated that the project would take fifteen months. In fact, by employing their captured POWs, it took just twelve months – and thousands of deaths. It needed a huge workforce and the Japanese accomplished this by sending overlapping labour parties of prisoners further and further north.

The Japanese began sending regular parties of POWs 'up country' from June 1942. No news about what happened there filtered back to Changi, and the Japanese encouraged the belief that conditions up country were better than in Singapore. In fact, the previous October, Harry had actually sent up country most of the painful feet cases and other cases of vitamin deficiency *in the hope that the change of air and food may cure them, for frankly there is no cure here*. They had heard that most of the travel was by truck or train, and although there was a two-day march at the end, the sick and lame would be allowed to travel by truck.

By April 1943 there were fewer than 10,000 prisoners left in Changi. Harry was assigned to F Force, a party of 7,000 British and Australian troops. It was the last group to go, and 30% of this party were classed as unfit either to march or work. Jim Bradley[5] said that most of the relatively fit men also had some kind of medical history since capitulation, and nearly all of them were reduced in strength owing to malnutrition.

However, everyone wanted to be included as they were issued with a list of all the reasons the move up country would be beneficial:

- The food situation in Singapore was difficult. A good canteen would be available in each camp and would be far better in the new place.
- This would not be a working party.
- They were going to a cooler climate in a pleasant hill place.
- The unfit men would have a better chance of recovery and good facilities for recreation.
- There would be no marching except for a short distance from the train to a nearby camp, and transport would be provided for baggage, and men unfit to march.

The group was encouraged to take band instruments, lighting sets, tools and their cooking gear, whilst they were told that gramophones, blankets, clothing and mosquito nets would be issued at the new camps. The force would include a medical party of about 350, with equipment for a central hospital of 400 patients and medical supplies for three months.

Every one was in a party mood and the Japanese seemed especially lenient during the preparations for the journey. At first neither Harry nor the Padre were included and relied on string-pulling and the influence of senior officers so that they too could benefit(!) from this new camp.

Harry and his team prepared carefully for the move. *Windmill, my medical orderly, has been working like a Trojan. He cleaned out a wooden medical box which he painted and stencilled with my name, and I have now converted it to my own use. He also made me a small, white, first aid box with all the necessary contents included. My haversack or pack he converted into a rucksack that clips on in front, and is adjustable. Two ammunition pouches that are stitched to the sides are very useful for holding toilet articles, etc.* Harry kept his basic medical kit canvas roll with him throughout. Apart from bandages and dressings, it was still intact and preserved with his other war memorabilia.

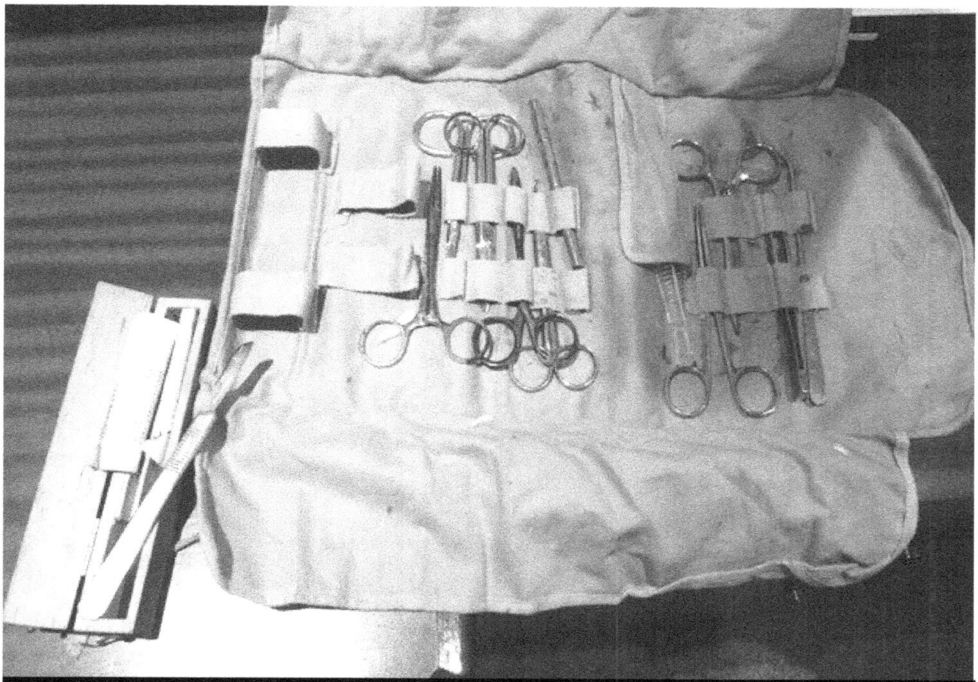

Harry's canvas medical kit

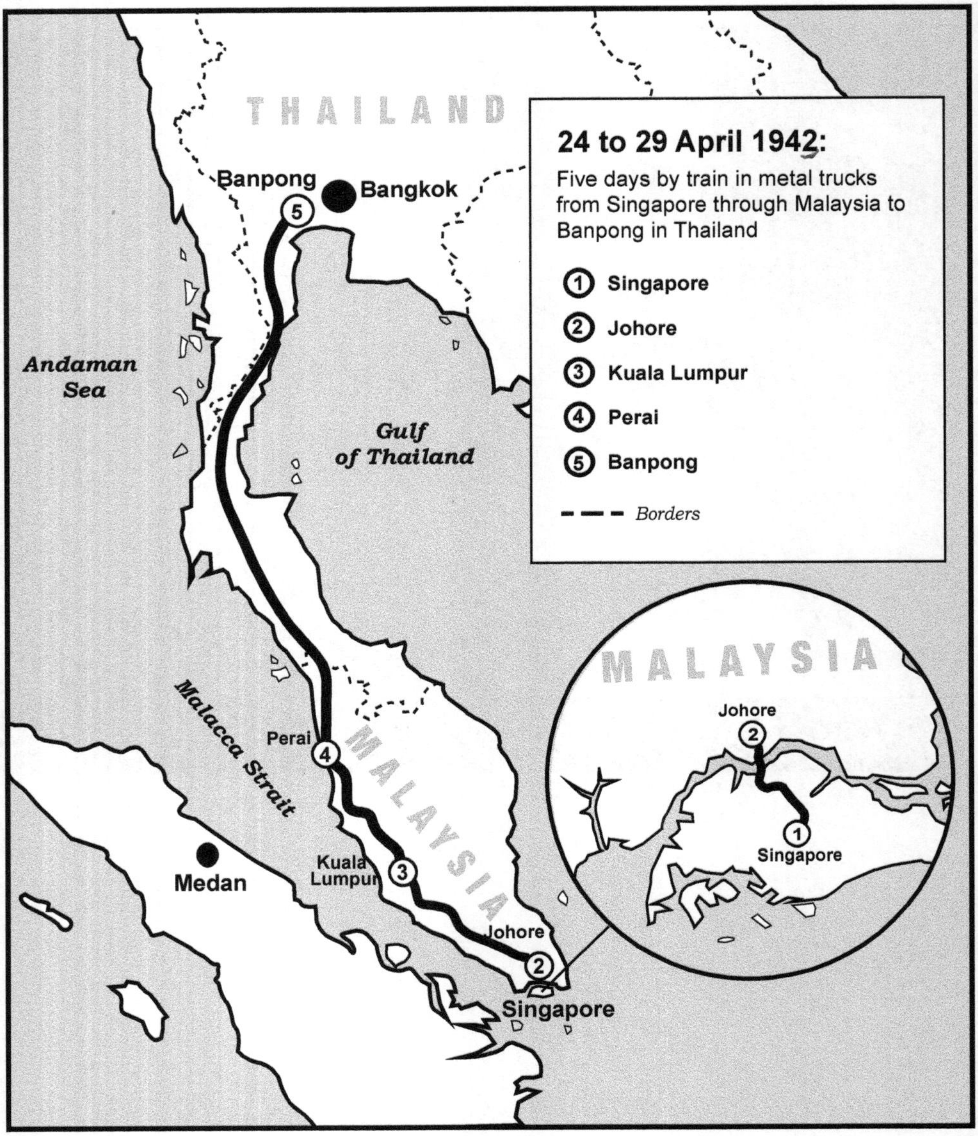
THAILAND
24 to 29 April 1942:
Five days by train in metal trucks from Singapore through Malaysia to Banpong in Thailand
1 Singapore
2 Johore
3 Kuala Lumpur
4 Perai
5 Banpong
Borders
Banpong
Bangkok
Andaman Sea
Gulf of Thailand
Malacca Strait
MALAYSIA
Perai
Kuala Lumpur
Medan
Johore
Singapore
MALAYSIA
Johore
Singapore

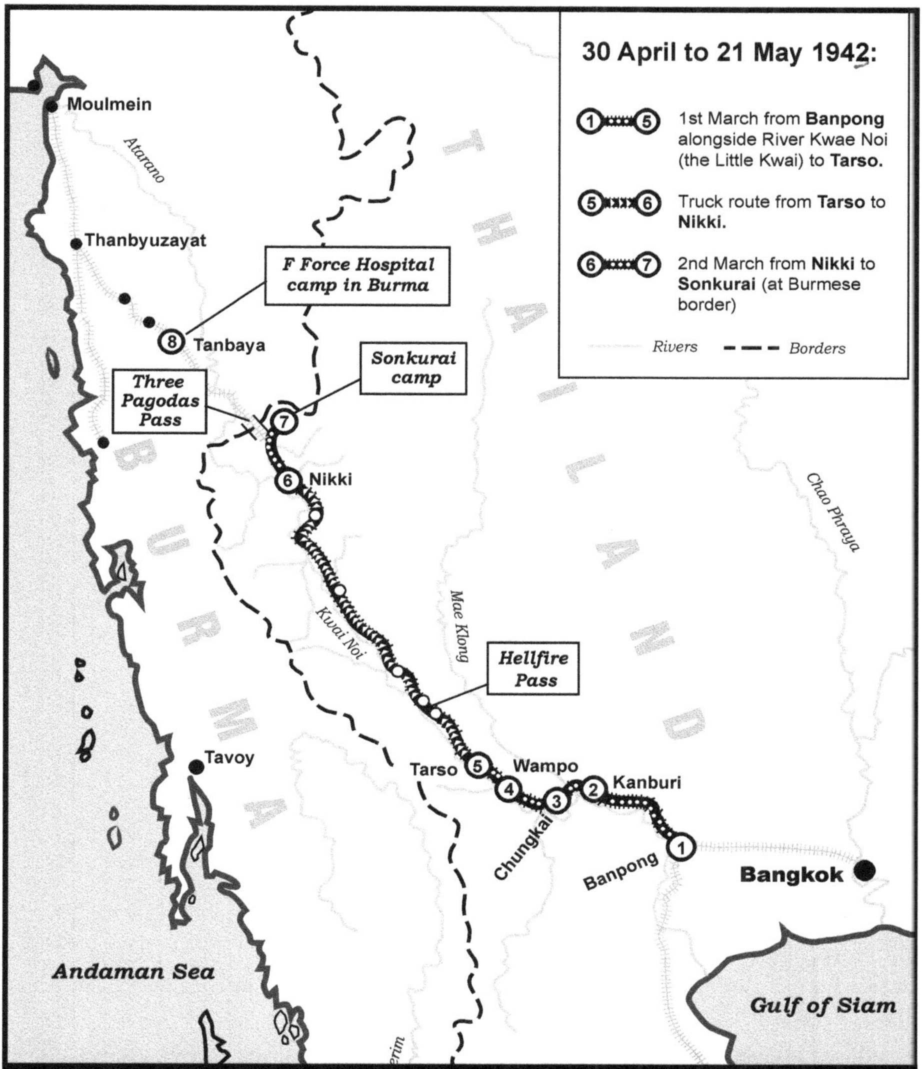

THE BURMA RAILWAY

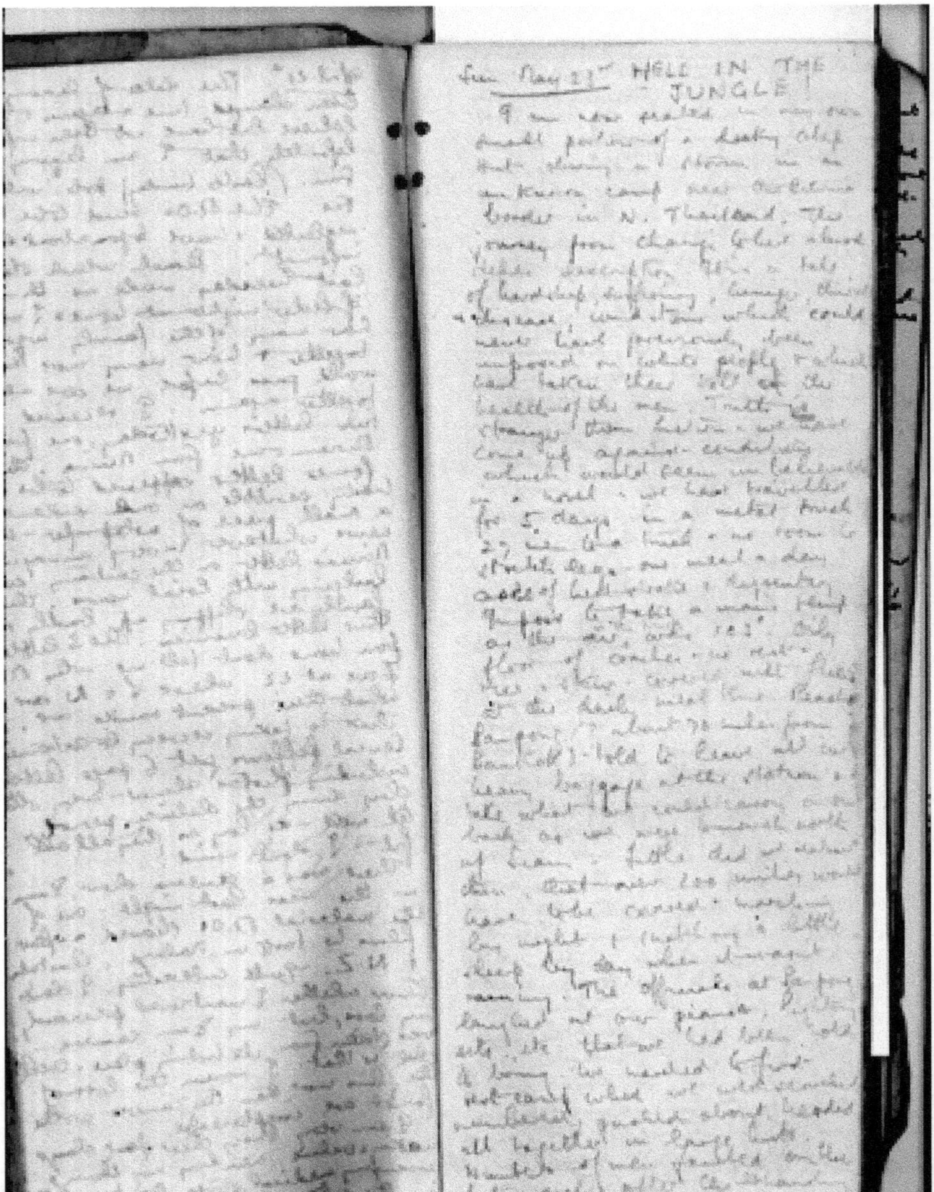
HELL IN THE
JUNGLE!

There is now a gap of over four weeks in Harry's diary. His next, very long, entry on 23rd May 1943 with a complete change of tone, was entitled

HELL IN THE JUNGLE

I am now seated in my own small portion of a leaky atap hut, during a storm in an unknown camp near the Burma border in northern Thailand. The journey from Changi to here almost defies description. It is a tale of hardship, suffering, hunger, thirst and disease, in conditions which could never have previously been imposed in a civilised society and which have taken their toll on the health of the men. Truth is stranger than fiction, and we have come up against conditions which would seem unbelievable in a novel.

The party left Singapore by train and travelled in metal rice trucks, about 30 men per truck. The trucks were totally enclosed and unventilated, apart from sliding doors in the centre of one side. Inside they were packed like sardines with no room to stretch their legs. There was no sanitation. Many of the POWs had acute dysentery, and in order to relieve themselves, had to hang out of the doors held by a chain. The walls of the truck were burning hot in the sun and there were numerous cases of heatstroke. Harry said *it was impossible to take a man's temperature as the air in the trucks was about 103°. The floors of the trucks were filthy and oily. There was no way we could rest.* Acute thirst was a major problem. They stopped once a day for a fly-covered rice meal. This journey lasted for five days, the last 24 hours without food or water.

They finally reached Banpong railway station. The Japanese officials laughed at all the gear they had been told to bring especially

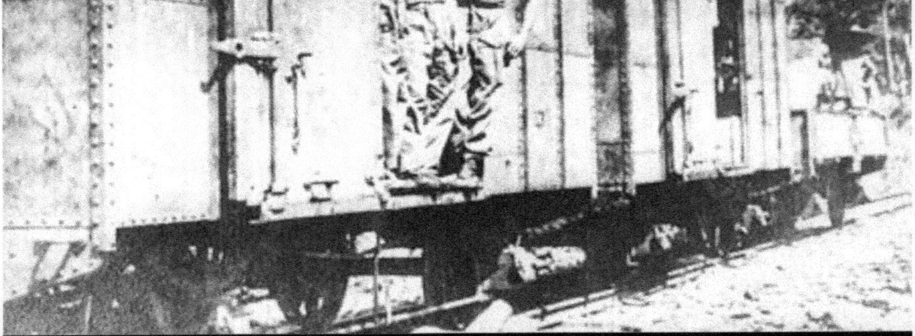

Metal rice truck

the pianos and lighting sets. They had to leave everything including precious medical equipment, taking only what they could carry in their backpacks for the long trek to northern Thailand. Vital medical supplies were distributed to those fit enough to carry them, but their backpacks were already very heavy.

The short march to the first camp after the gruelling train journey was too much for the many unfit men who were just out of hospital in Changi. *We were searched, numbered, pushed about, and herded altogether in large huts. Numbers of men fainted on the short march after the exhausting rail journey*. The realisation of the truth about 'good rest camps' was starting to hit home.

They had one night's rest, but it was impossible to sleep, before beginning their 200-mile march. This would have been a problem for fit men in reasonable territory, but it was horrendous in dense mountainous jungle and the monsoon climate. They marched by night as it was too hot during the day, carrying everything on their backs, eventually discarding the heavier items as help was needed to carry the sick. They toiled through pitch blackness. It wasn't surprising that men fell off the mountain sides and bridges in the dark and there were many fractured arms and legs from falls. Stragglers were attacked by marauding Thai natives.

Each night march covered about 15 to 20 miles. This may not sound much, but when only two-thirds of the men are fit when leaving Changi, exhausted by a long, stifling train journey, having to carry all their kit on their backs, struggling through jungle paths and swamps, and often through tropical storms on very poor rations, with diarrhoea rife, struggling on night after night, with blistered feet, very few medical supplies – all these throw a different light on the picture. At the rest camps, there were no tents. One just had to find shade under a tree. If it rained, one waited, shivering, for it to stop, and then build a fire to dry out one's clothing.

I was medical officer in charge of my train party and marched at the tail end of the column which often straggled out for several hundred yards. Consequently, at a halt, I treated the stragglers and by the time I caught up with the main group, the halt was almost over. I was exhausted assisting the sick, lame and the weary, supporting them, carrying stretchers, and helping with their kit, in spite of my own kit which I had to carry. My mental and physical condition can be imagined as I struggled on through a tropical storm, through water, swirling and rushing waist-high on two occasions. One of my shoes was torn off, so I discarded the other one and completed the journey barefooted. Every step was agony.

Meagre rations consisted of rice and water. Rest camps had no tents, just clearings in the jungle. They tried to find shade from the sun or shelter from the rain under trees. Many hundreds died on the way up country, mostly from malnutrition, malaria and dysentery. At one rest camp, Harry himself was classed as unfit to march further by a Japanese MO. *He was very strict and examined all the men who were left behind who were marked unfit to travel. He sent on cases of diarrhoea, dysentery, septic and blistered feet, etc. It made my blood boil to see the weary men with large, swollen and septic feet, infected blisters and ulcers, having to hobble away at night. I can feel for them, as I know what they went through.*

Although unwell himself, Harry was needed to look after the sick at this camp. After five days, he was allowed to continue the next stage of the journey by truck, accompanying the sick.

Travelling by truck sounds good, but going on a heavy five-tonner through a Thai jungle, up and down very steep slopes, across dangerous swaying bamboo bridges which broke under the wheels, clinging on to the baggage on which we were so precariously balanced, bumping incessantly up and down till all parts of our bodies were sore, seeing the back wheels skid on the slippery edge of a precipice as we looked down from the truck straight onto the water fifty or sixty feet below and going across the sides of a quarry on a rough road made out of shifting stone, pushing the truck several miles when it broke down, climbing off and on to push it out of muddy ruts, keeping back the shifting machinery, redhot from the sun, blistering our backs and hands, seeing two trucks overturn going over narrow bridges and dropping into the valley below – that's what driving by truck meant.

Harry's green medical case miraculously survived unscathed after being hurled twice into a ravine. His 2-volt battery lamp, a dinner plate and a mirror, did not break, which was good testimony to the packer.

Harry then continued the journey on foot. F Force had to trudge past many work camps, when they learned there was cholera in the camp. G P Adams[10] said that people in these camps would watch F Force plodding past. 'However sorry we may have been for ourselves, our hearts could bleed for the unfortunates of F Force who passed by our camp for days on end. All were tired and worn.'

At one staging camp, cholera was discovered too late to stop it spreading. The ground was covered with infected faeces, but the Japanese refused to lend spades to the British officers who wanted to remove this dreadful health hazard, and said 'use your hands'. Inoculations were feverishly given, and all the troops were moved out to another camp. Harry tried to isolate the sick by moving them away from the camp into a clearing in the jungle where there were numerous sandflies and mosquitoes. Alone there to look after the sick, while other parties came and went, he had to wait three days with no covering or medical supplies until a truck came to transport them to the next staging camp.

He found that this experience would repeat itself throughout the long trek. It was expected that each succeeding medical officer took over the MI Room for one day before continuing the march. *The MI rooms in the rest camps were hastily improvised shelters, and often had no covering at all. The MOs left behind to look after the sick had a difficult job with no supplies and very few facilities for treatment. In most of the camps I did my own sick parade, often very large, while the rest of the men and officers were sleeping.*

Jim Bradley[5] wrote about the work of the doctors on the march:

> 'First [the doctors] would be called to a casualty falling back at the rear of the column, and next they would be wanted up front. When we arrived at our staging camps,

> completely without shelter, we would throw ourselves on the ground and perhaps take off our boots if we dared …. The doctors, however, held sick parades, attending to men's blistered and burnt feet, and doing what they could for the sick and dying. They took little time to rest themselves, but I believe they received scant recognition for all they did, except in the gratitude which showed on the faces of all those whom they helped.'

Harry said frequently that their captivity brought out the best and worst in men. *On one or two occasions, Major Barber who was OC our party managed to stop a truck for the lame and sick. There was a disgusting scramble for lifts by fit men. At times like this, I was very disappointed by the behaviour of some of the men who were very selfish, so that towards the end of the journey, in spite of the difficulties, I ceased to have much sympathy for them.*

He would grab a few minutes respite whenever he could. *I used to have difficulty sleeping on the hard ground or a strange bed. The few minutes rest we had at each halt would see me throw myself down where I stood, on the muddy road, and fall fast asleep till awakened all too soon, stiff and weary, to continue the agony. I made the mistake originally of trying to take too much kit, and suffered from the heavy pack on my back. It felt much lighter when the blanket and mosquito net were discarded.*

They were given one small meal a day, but it left them extremely hungry and thirsty. *Fortunately the Nip guards allowed us to descend at most of the stations and buy food. The hot sweet coffee and hard-boiled eggs that I bought at dawn at Alastare will always be in my memory as one of the most welcome meals I have ever had. We stuffed ourselves with papaya, bananas and eggs at each halt, so we managed to keep going. We were able to wash when we stopped by a river. At one place we had to do PT!*

It upset Harry greatly that the weakened men were expected to clear the tracks for the troops. *It pained me to see the thin bodies of men heaving stones from the side of the quarry and they are expected to keep going on poor rations. How they can do this hard work is beyond my comprehension.*

He said that on the whole they were treated fairly well by the guards who accompanied them. *It was the Nips at the halts who beat the men and made officers do general fatigues and cookhouse duties. Beatings were all too common. I am looking forward to the day when it will all be repaid with interest.*

Some five weeks after leaving Changi after yet another night march: we *were certainly glad to reach our final destination after so many so-called 'final' ones. And so ended the long and weary trek through 200 miles of wild jungle to our new home where we may stay till the end of the war. The condition of the men as they arrived beggars description – no boots, tattered clothes, sunken cheeks, unshaven faces. It was often impossible to recognise old friends. However the relief of being able to lie down and sleep at night surpasses all else.*

Chapter Eight

Railway

You can't eat a cigarette case

They had reached Sonkurai in Thailand, near the Three Pagodas Pass, and Harry stayed in this area for ten weeks. It was a sea of mud at the height of the monsoon. They slept on platforms made of split bamboo with a space of 2ft wide for each man.

The POWs had no running water, no soap, no toothpaste or toilet paper. They sold whatever surplus clothes and possessions they had to local natives to get money to buy food. Many of the men were reduced to wearing just loincloths.

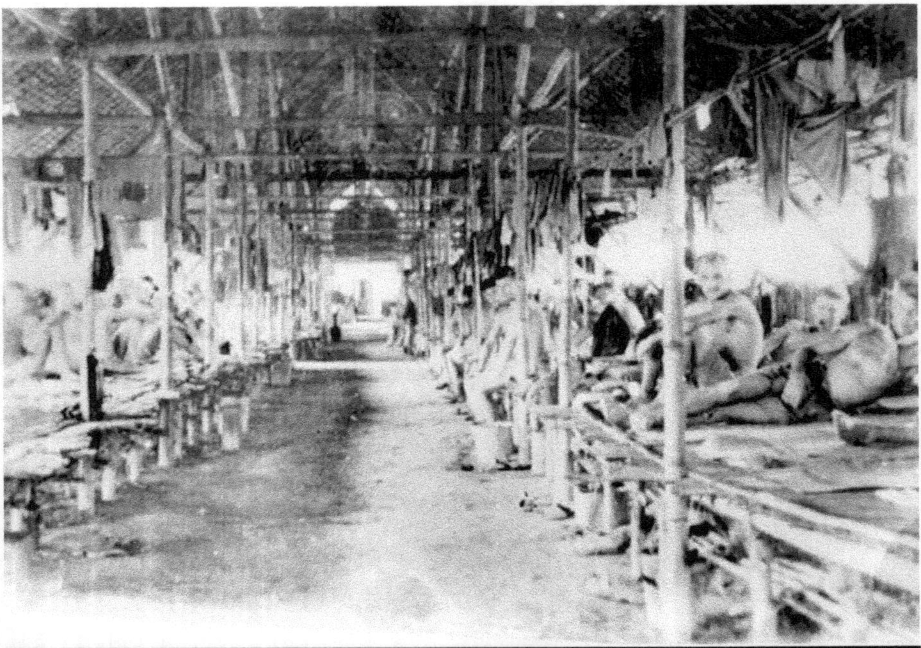

Sleeping platforms

In the Yorkshire Television documentary[1] Harry said he sold a gold filling from his teeth plus precious items he had managed to save up to this point: his gold watch (which had been a graduation present from his father), his wallet and a gold cigarette case: 'you couldn't eat a cigarette case very well. My thoughts were only for survival.'

On one occasion, Harry was the only 'fit' person and he collected the wherewithal to buy eggs. He bought about six dozen, a supply which he intended to eke out over a number of days for his sick patients. Walking back to the camp, his heart sank when a Japanese guard on a passing railway truck forced him at bayonet point onto the train. As he neared the camp and was able to see smoke from the fires, the guard, with an evil grin, caused the train to pick up speed. Harry had no option but to jump backwards from the truck, trying in vain to protect his precious bundle of eggs. That night many POWs benefited from an enormous omelette made with the eggs, including the broken shells and bits of fluff from inside his pack.

The captives were grateful to the brave men who, at risk of being shot if discovered, had carried radio parts in their packs during the long trek through the jungle. Using the battery the Japanese guards let Harry have for lighting, they were able to keep up to date with news of the war in Europe.

The construction of the Burma Railway was a huge project made much harder as the Japanese provided no heavy construction equipment. The prisoners built the railway entirely by hand. They broke the ground with pickaxes and shovels. They moved earth with buckets and bamboo-and-burlap litters. Stone-crushing for ballast was done with hammers. To bore holes in hard rock they used iron drills and sledgehammers.

The men had to work under unbelievably terrible conditions, being treated like slaves with daily beatings using wire whips and bamboo

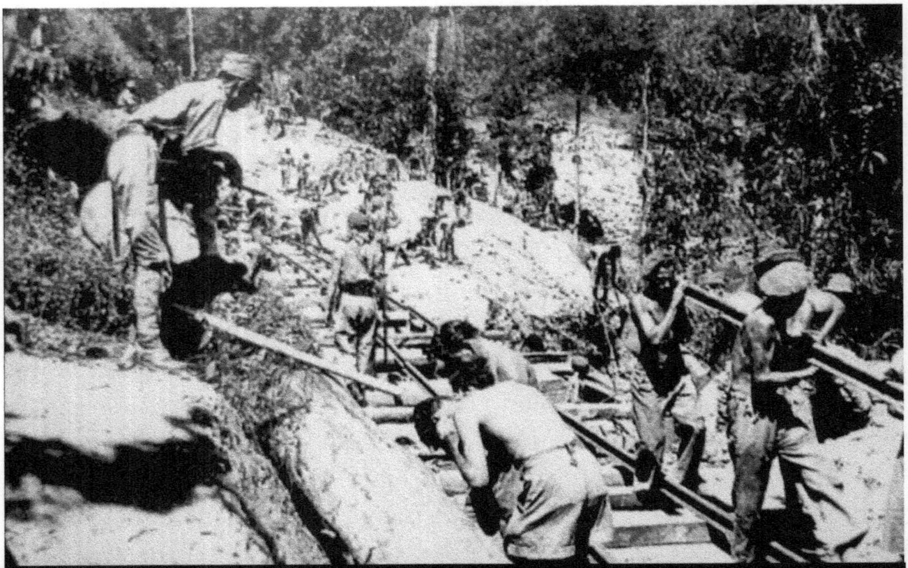

Hellfire Pass

sticks. One punishment was being made to stand holding a heavy rock above their head for hours in the full sun with a sharpened bamboo stick propped against the prisoner's back. If he wavered, as inevitably happened, the bamboo stick pierced his skin. If he dropped the rock before an unspecified moment, he was beaten. Some guards just threw rocks at the prisoners for fun. When the guards finally accepted that a prisoner was too ill to work on the railway, they would stop his rations as he was now no use to them. These men were kept alive solely on rice shared by 'active' men from their own rations.

Because of the lack of hygiene, minimal food rations and slave labour conditions, the POWs suffered and died from a huge number of tropical diseases. Sanitary conditions were appalling, and there was no dedicated MI accommodation. However, after Harry had treated one of

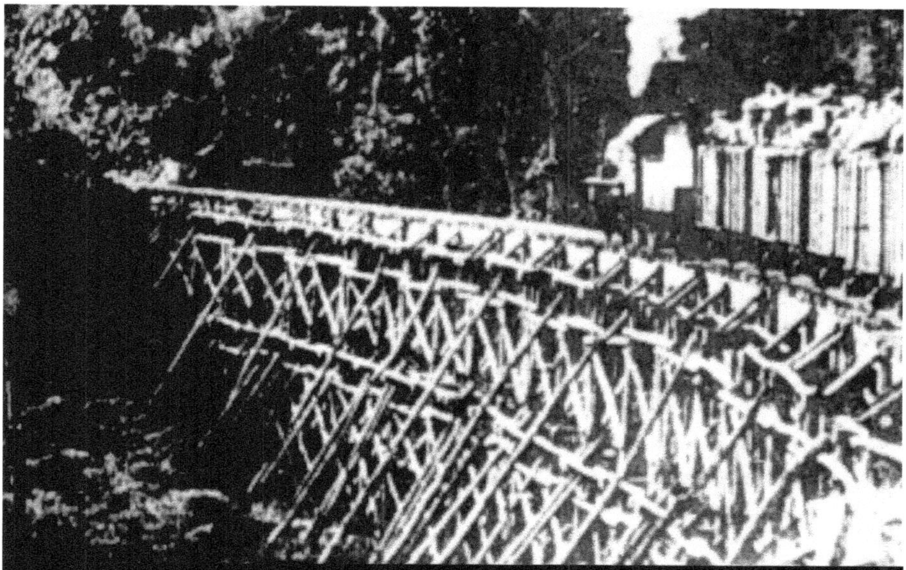

Burma Railway

the Japanese officers, he was allowed to use a hut as an MI room which he said was a godsend.

He sometimes worked a 24-hour day, with very little in the way of medical treatment. Cholera was a major problem. It had been brought to the camps by Burmese labourers who were conscripted by the Japanese. Harry said the curse had followed them all the way up country, affecting the Australian and British POWs alike. Every day he logged the number of cholera cases and subsequent deaths. *The number of cases is increasing daily, and we are holding conferences, etc. A hygiene officer has been appointed, and everything possible is being done. At first the isolation place was an unroofed small hut in which patients lay soaking and froze to death. Now we have a roofed isolation place and the two far ends of the big hut are used for hospital accommodation.*

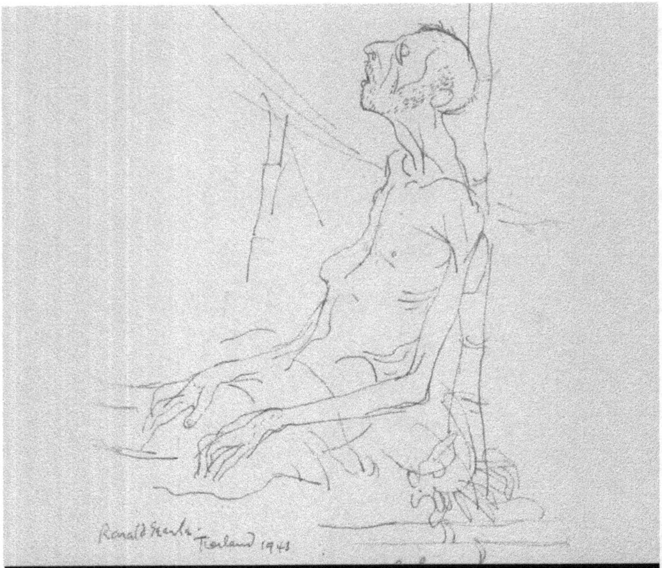

Ronald Searle: man dying of cholera

At one point he was caring single-handedly for up to four hundred cholera patients and he estimated that one man in ten died of cholera in the camp. It is clear from the YTV documentary[1] made nearly 70 years later that these scenes were still vividly remembered: 'Doing a ward round in a cholera ward, it is indescribable. They're just writhing in agony, vomiting, they've got diarrhoea, their faces are shrunken and they're just skin and bones. It was such a painful end for them. They wanted something to help them, but I had nothing to give them.'

The only relief that could be provided was rehydration, giving cooled boiled water via what Harry called Heath Robinson contraptions, contrived from his stethoscope tube attached to a needle made from bamboo. His diary entries during this time are filled with descriptions

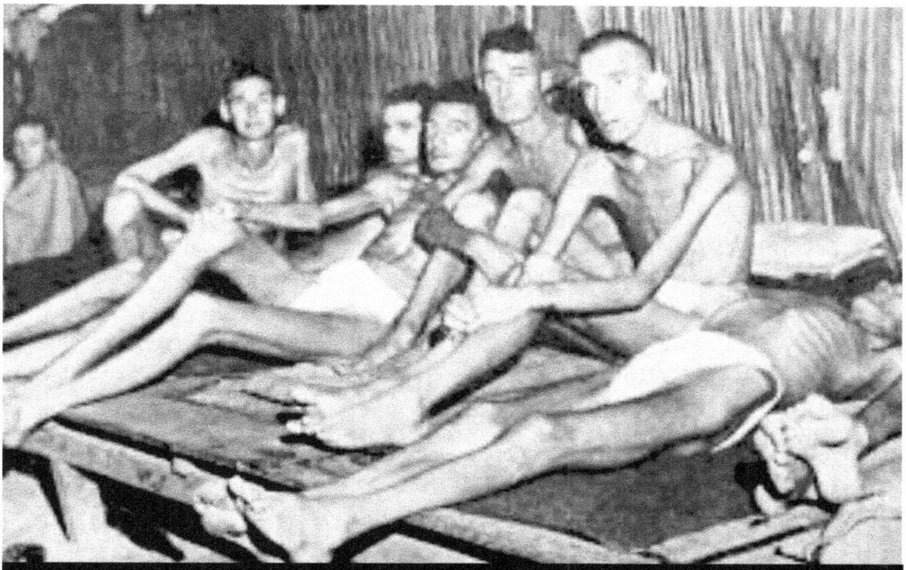

POWs at the Burma Railway camp. Living skeletons

of this nightmare period. *It looks like a scene from a film, completely unreal. Groans and cries are the only noises to break the silence. About nine corpses lay outside covered with blankets and groundsheets, and a little distance away, the smoke of the pyre where the corpses are burning could be seen. We have a gruesome job here, burning the dead cholera patients. It is a terrible, tragic end to die of disease in a jungle camp like this. I have never been so weary in all my life. I just drag one foot after the other, leaning on a stick.*

Another condition that affected many of the prisoners was a tropical ulcer of the legs caused by infected scratches from cut bamboo, and it spread rapidly. With the right treatment, this is not a fatal disease, but the doctors had nothing that would help. *I saw my former batman,*

Windmill, today. He is in the ulcer ward, and looks a wreck of his former vigorous self. He pleaded with me with tears in his eyes for his leg to be taken off, but as he is such a bad operative risk, I understand it will not be done. He says the pain is terrific, twenty-four hours a day, and at night he is afraid of losing his reason. What a terrible thing a tropical ulcer is. Amputation is the only treatment and relief, and the post-operative mortality is very high. Windmill did have his amputation, but died a few days later. Harry mourned this tragic end for a healthy young lad.

Every day brought fresh cases of other diseases including malaria, dysentery, beriberi, various fevers and even smallpox and typhus. He had a number of diphtheria cases which he found very upsetting. *One feels so helpless. With these cases there are no antitoxins, just rest, and the men are choking to a slow and painful death.* Not surprisingly many of the MOs were ill themselves, and on one occasion Harry did a ward round carried on a stretcher after he had fainted.

It really distressed him that there was so little he could do for the sick. His diary records the daily number of deaths from disease and malnutrition at the railway work camps. The Japanese guards demanded a minimum number of men to work on the railway each day. It became more and more difficult to find this number as the death toll increased daily but the guards were relentless, driving out everyone they thought could put in even the smallest amount of work. The doctors had the terrible task of deciding which of the sick men were least sick.

In the YTV programme[1] Harry said 'In the morning, a certain number, say 60, had to go out on the working party. If I couldn't find 60 fit people I used to tell them. It didn't make any difference. They would go along saying "you, you, you and you, you and you". I'd say they can't go, they're too ill. The bayonets would come out and I knew what would happen. They'd be carried back dead.' As the Japanese had huge numbers of prisoners, the death toll was immaterial to them.

Jim Bradley[5] greatly admired the way the doctors worked under such appalling conditions.

> 'The one I remember with particular affection was Dr Harry Silman who worked ceaselessly for the benefit of all. I had known him so well in Changi, as he was one of those with whom I had sat and talked on the roof of our barrack block at night. He was always cheerful, despite our circumstances.'

Inevitably, friends and colleagues of Harry died during this time. Each death was a tragedy. *We heard yesterday that John Excell died. It was a terrible shock. He was the life and soul of any mess. He had started designing my house which he called Bedside Manor! ... Sgt Armstrong, my medical sergeant from the beginning, died a few days ago from dysentery. He had put up a hard fight. I was very sad, and I was with him when he died peacefully.*

The cause of death was not always illness or disease. Some could not cope with the sheer effort of staying alive. 'There was a warrant officer who was 6'3". A fine fellow. He really had nothing wrong with him, except that he didn't want to keep on living. When he took to his bed I used to sit and chat to him. I took his wallet out, and showed him the photo of his wife and children. I said now surely you want to go back. It was the most amazing thing. He just faded away and died.'[1]

At the end of July Harry was moved to Tanbaya in Burma, where a hospital camp had been set up for 2,000 patients. There were echoes of their horrendous march up country. *We left number 2 camp on Friday, 30th July in pouring rain and marched to number 5 camp where we stopped overnight. We left there at 3.30 am and marched in pitch blackness for ten kilometres. Many men fell into rivers, ditches, etc, and some men lost their kit. I was unable to see clearly in the dark, and had to hold on to the man in front like a blind man. We trucked to Kandoo, and then by train to Ronshi. We marched from there as a bridge had been swept away by the storm, and we arrived at Tanbaya where the hospital is stationed.*

Conditions were slightly better here. To begin with the Japanese guards *were a nasty bunch who led us a hell of a life*, but later they got a new Japanese administration *consisting mostly of kindly-looking elderly Japs who are in stark contrast to their predecessors. They left us strictly alone, increased our food, and generally allowed us everything we asked for.*

Many of the medical staff there had malaria, and it was sometimes hard to find sufficient people to carry out essential tasks. Patients were brought in, usually in the middle of the night, so fires for the bath-house and illuminating flares needed to be lit. They had to lift the helpless patients off the trucks and carry them into the camp hospital.

The condition of the patients was terrible after a nightmare journey for three days in open trucks and trains, often in pouring rain. Several died on the journey, and some were brought here dead. This morning, out of a party of 114 that left no. 2 camp, 14 died on the way here and were buried en route, and 6 were brought in dead. It seems to me to be a criminal act to send these dying men on a long journey for no purpose at all, and sending no fit men or medical orderlies with them. It is absolutely amazing.

Men arrived daily, barely alive with every bone showing. Harry said that even the Japanese were amazed when they saw these living skeletons.

When Harry first arrived, the food was quite adequate, but although the number of patients went up, the rations did not go up accordingly. After a week, the total number had increased from the first group of 60 patients to 1,600, and the accommodation was extremely crowded. It was obvious that the food would have to improve to save lives. Gradually conditions got better. Stores of mosquito nets, blankets and cooking utensils were sent in, and much-needed items of clothing. There were increased supplies of food, but it did not stop the rising death tally in the hospital – over 200 after just 18 days.

Harry himself was ill again, this time from a type of malaria that also had symptoms of tropical typhus. The only treatment available was quinine, but it seemed to help. He found it difficult to sleep as his nights were very much disturbed *by ants in their millions who climb up the posts at the back of the bed, and scatter in search of food. Ants in the hair are enough to make anyone go mad. I have killed thousands, but it makes no appreciable difference to the numbers.*

He was upset to hear news of the death of the last man from the concert party which left Changi with F Force. The atrocious working conditions on the railway meant that, at best, there were just a few attempts to have sing-alongs round campfires. Every single account written by Japanese POWs pays tribute to the entertainers who kept up morale in the most unbelievably difficult circumstances.

By the end of November, the death toll in the hospital in Tanbaya had reached 640. The railway had now been completed and most of the doctors and surviving patients were to leave for Singapore. A small medical and administrative staff were left behind in Burma to look after about 250 men who were too sick to move, but the rest were sent on, by the railway built by the prisoners, to Kanburi. This was not a comfortable journey. It took four days, and they were crowded 33 to a truck. However, at the station they were greeted by *a large bevy of female vendors of eggs, bananas, coffee etc, and we indulged in an orgy of spending. Up until then we had very little opportunity of spending our Thai money.*

Finally they travelled back to Singapore. They were taken from the station to Changi by truck in the early hours of 21st December 1943, Harry's 33rd birthday. The clock chimed midnight as they arrived into the silent dark streets, and Harry told his fellow officers the significance of the date. Immediately they started singing Happy Birthday, and the Japanese driver stopped the truck to see what was going on. He could not understand why they seemed so happy, and Harry said the driver clearly thought the British were quite mad!

F Force proved to be the most ill-fated of all the parties. They were sent to the most northerly of all the working camps on the railway. Out of the original 7,000 men who went up country, 3,800 died. The treatment of the men whilst building the Burma Railway was the biggest sustained POW atrocity of the Pacific War.

Chapter Nine

Liberation

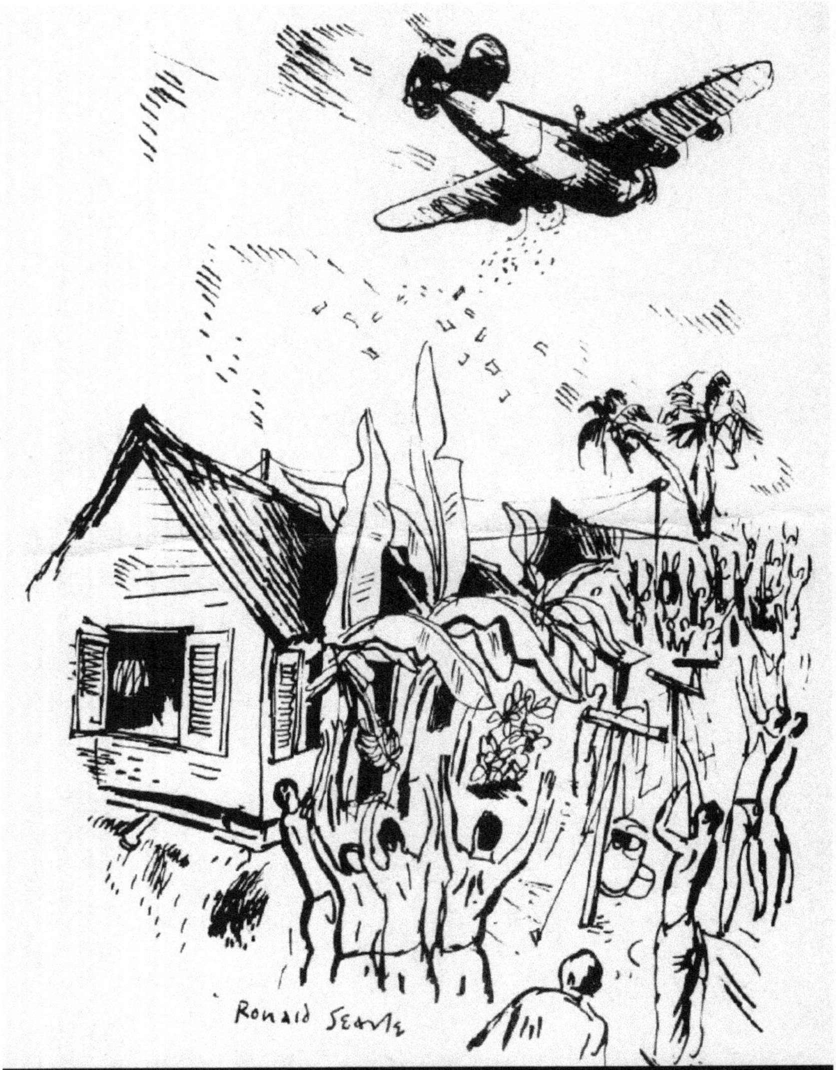

Ronald Searle: Plane dropping pamphlets announcing the end of the war

The event we have been looking forward to so eagerly

Once the prisoners were back in Changi, life became more normal. Their old quarters were being converted into an aerodrome, so the POWs were housed temporarily in huts and houses before being moved into the civilian Changi Gaol while the civilians, who had previously been housed there, were relocated to the Sime Road camp. A thousand British prisoners were crammed inside the gaol. *Initially there is a depressing atmosphere about the place which takes some time to get used to. Two high walls surrounding the gaol are guarded by Nips, all windows are enclosed with bars and wire mesh and one gets a feeling of being hemmed in. I feel it particularly after the open air comfort of the last billet.*

A few weeks later, Harry was reaccommodated into one of the huts just outside the gaol. It was also very cramped, the officers *lying cheek by jowl and some are double berthing in order to give themselves more floor space.* There was a spate of remarkable orders with pernickety details about the dressing of beds, and instructions that all clothes lines had to run north-south. Harry had no idea if these were at the instigation of the Japanese or British. Later he was moved once more into one of three houses known as Harley Street, as they were used for sick officers and the MOs. Here they had more space, and gardens where they could grow vegetables.

Although the rations continued to be poor and there were still incidents of torture and deprivation, conditions were never as bad as those up country. The POWs settled into a routine, renewing the Changi University and the wonderful shows which kept up the men's morale. Harry praised an excellent production of Hay Fever which had a professional actor as the main lead.

He attended a couple of lectures given by an Italian officer on modern submarine warfare. *It is a strange state of affairs when we hear one of our former enemies talk about his part in the undersea warfare against our shipping and an amazing thing to hear the cheers at the end for a man who recently was helping to sink our merchant fleet.* This reference to an Italian officer in Changi may seem quite puzzling, but there were two Italian submarines in Singapore when Italy capitulated in September 1943. The crews were given the choice of pro- or anti-Mussolini allegiance, and about a third chose the latter, in spite of the probable consequence of imprisonment.

Harry still read in his leisure time, and played a nightly game of bridge. He took pleasure in a good debate and went to one entitled 'If we want peace, we must prepare for war'. The motion was carried.

Harry had built up a collection of artwork given to him by fellow POWs. Typical of the British sense of humour is a drawing entitled the Decline & Fall of a Tin Hat. It chronicles the imaginary stages of alternative uses of the soldier's tin hat, finishing as a receptacle for stools held by a skeletal prisoner outside a laboratory.

The prisoners were allowed to go down to the sea which was very beneficial. They not only welcomed the opportunity to go swimming, but could also bring back wood for the fires and coconuts for the mess.

While F Force was up country, there was a daring escape by ten men who hoped to tell the world about the brutal conditions on the railway. Only four survived, including Harry's friend Jim Bradley. *They are very lucky to be alive after their most amazing adventures. They had to hack their way through thick jungle and climb high ranges of mountains daily. This slowed their speed and they ran short of food, and*

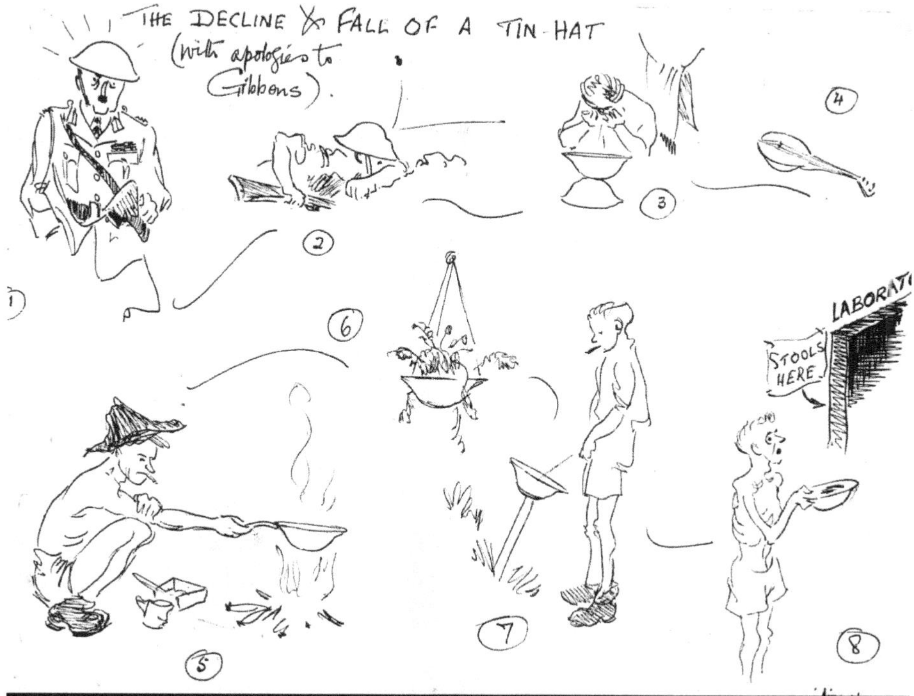

Decline and Fall of a Tin Hat by T A T Hickham

for the last three weeks of their journey they starved. Four officers died, one by one, and were left – a tragic end – somewhere in the jungle. They built a raft when they came to a river but the current was strong and carried them over rocks and falls and finally it smashed in midstream. They were flung into the water and had to swim for their lives. They later saw some native hunters up a canal who looked after them for a few days but finally gave them up to the Japs.

The survivors were brought back for interrogation and trial. It was expected that they would be tortured or executed or both, but miraculously they were sentenced to nine or ten years penal servitude in Outram Road Gaol. This was infamous as a place of starvation and terror, but they were all released on grounds of ill health after a couple of months, and were sent back to hospital in Changi.

Harry was very happy that he could visit Jim Bradley and the other escapees in hospital. In fact, Jim Bradley credited his survival to Harry who, before the escape, had given him some sulphonamides to treat two small tropical ulcers. He put these on each ulcer, binding them with mosquito netting and thus averted a potential life-threatening deterioration.

An unpleasant incident happened to Padre Cordingly during this period. He had to spend two days in a pit handcuffed to an acting sergeant for carrying letters from one camp to another containing alleged news. This was not the first such episode for the Padre. While they were on the railway in Thailand he had offered a similar service. Since most men there had no clothes but a tattered loin cloth and he owned a pair of shorts, he had been given scribbled notes to pass on, asking for news of friends. Unfortunately he and an Indian doctor with the party were stopped and searched, and accused of being spies. They were handcuffed to each other and thrown into a pit. While it was still dark, a young Japanese guard lowered a ladder into the pit, and offered them sweet tea and two bananas. The Padre was released the next day, but there is no doubt the young soldier would have been executed if his humanitarian action had been discovered.

Harry was kept busy with his medical duties. Malaria was rife, with a shortage of quinine, and there were still many cases of dysentery and stomatitis. Their diet continued to be very short of vitamin B, especially because now there were no rice polishings, so there were increased numbers of vitamin-deficient diseases such as beriberi. Harry

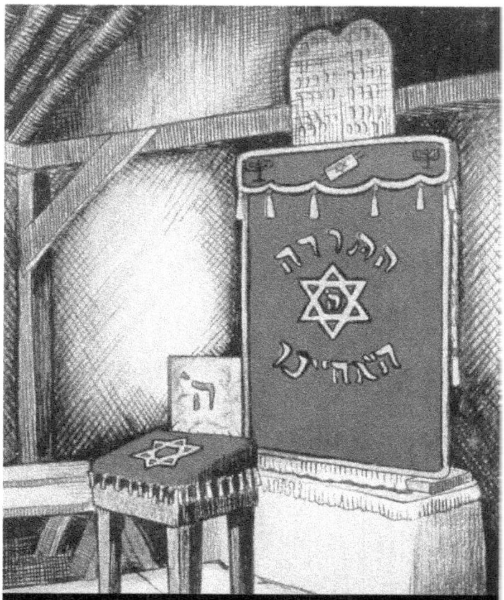

Ohel Jacob Synagogue

himself had spells of poor health, including an acute attack of bacterial dysentery which left him feeling really ill for several days.

Very gradually conditions improved. The Japanese allowed them more Red Cross parcels, sharing one parcel between seven men. Harry said the American parcels had a good variety of tins containing health foods and vitamins. They also received batches of old mail which had accumulated in their absence up country – Harry was given eleven letters, all about a year old.

In August 1944 the Japanese provided materials to build a small synagogue which was named Ohel Jacob. *Last Saturday night I was a spectator of a rather unique ceremony – the dedication of Ohel Jacob the recently built shul in the gaol. Everything was built and prepared by the boys themselves. A representation of the tablets above the ark was painted realistically and a (suitably) decorated curtain hung in front of an imaginary ark.* This fulfilled the need for a permanent place of worship. It became a haven of peace in what was at the time a very overcrowded prison.

Harry celebrated his 34th birthday on December 21st 1944 with *a pie made of tapioca root, tomatoes (own grown) and 2 tins of veg soup and numerous extras. Ted – our Messing officer – made it himself and made a jolly good job of it. It was very tasty and we all felt happily replete at the end.* He said he kept hoping it would be his last birthday as a POW, but had stopped speculating about the future.

The Japanese cancelled a grand fairground, planned by the officers to celebrate Christmas, but the POWs did eat well. *Xmas passed as usual with the traditional stuffing of oneself. There was an enormous meal on Xmas night after a big tiffin and tea and consequently most of it was left. Some including the Xmas cake was eaten the following day. I think that in a POW camp where rations are poor, the extra food should be spread over a few days and ease the shock of going back to ordinary meals.*

Over 300 toys were made by the POWs and sent over to Sime Road camp for the children of the civilian prisoners.

In August 1945 the long-circulating rumours that the war in the Far East was ending were confirmed. This is Harry's final diary entry:

August 25th 1945.
The event we have been looking forward to so eagerly for the past 3½ years has now taken place and with a suddenness that surprised us all. Early morning of August 11th found most of the camp up, in little groups discussing the rumour that the Emperor had agreed to accept the terms of the Potsdam conference. When this was confirmed later in the day we began to make plans for celebrations and an early evacuation.

Most of the tapioca root in the gardens was pulled up and consumed over 3 days and our little conclave Dixie, Doug Walker, John McNeath and I had 3 successive evening parties when we opened our reserve tins of food (fish and meat), condensed milk and emergency chocolate. We also pulled up all our greens, roots etc and had continuous food orgies. But day succeeded day and we still had Japanese roll call parades and had to salute the Nips and generally carried on as previously. This was a bit of an anti-climax and we had a bit of a shock when the local commander said that he intended to fight on and defend the island. However an order from the Emperor to cease fire ultimately reached the island after 10 days of ups and downs of spirits.

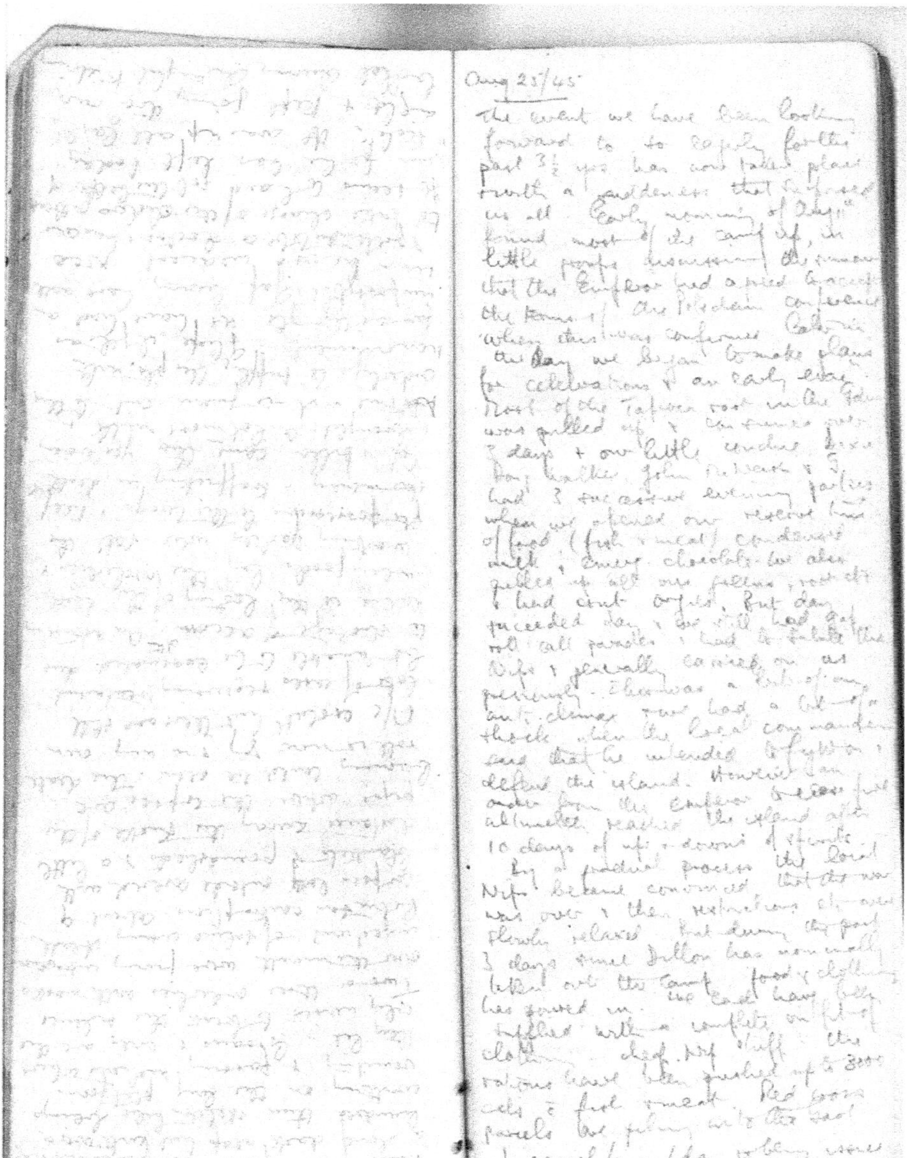
Aug 25/45
The event we have been looking forward to so keenly for the past 3½ yrs has now taken place with a suddenness that surprised us all. Early morning of Aug 11th found most of the camp up, in little groups discussing the rumour that the Emperor had agreed to accept the terms of the Potsdam conference. [illegible] this was confirmed. Later in the day we began to make plans for celebrations & an early exit. Most of the Tapioca root in the garden was pulled up & [illegible] 3 days & our little [illegible] Ray Walker, John [illegible] & I had 3 successive evening parties when we opened our reserve tins of food (fish & meat) condensed milk & emergency chocolate. We also pulled up all our pillows, root etc & had stout [illegible]. But day succeeded day & we still had got roll call parades & had to salute the Nips & generally carried on as previously. There was a bit of an anti-climax & we had a bit of a shock when the local commander said that he intended to fight on & defend the island. However an order from the Emperor to cease fire ultimately reached the island after 10 days of ups & downs of spirits.
By a gradual process the local Nips became convinced that the war was over & their restrictions on us slowly relaxed but during the past 3 days since Dillon has nominally taken over the camp food & clothing has poured in. We each have been supplied with a complete outfit of clothing [illegible] Nip stuff. The rations have been pushed up to 3000 cals & fish & meat. Red Cross parcels are going in to the tune of $\frac{1}{20}$ parcel/man/day, [illegible] & cigarettes etc at frequent intervals. Nussbaum got [illegible]

By a gradual process the local Nips became convinced that the war was over and then restrictions etc were slowly relaxed. But during the past 3 days since Dillon has nominally taken over the camp, food and clothing has poured in. We each have been supplied with a complete outfit of clothing – cheap Nip stuff – the rations have been pushed up to 3000 calories and fish and meat. Red Cross parcels are piling into the Gaol. 1/20 parcel per man per day is being issued and cigarettes etc at frequent intervals. Nussbaum put on a party in the shool (synagogue) *and a thanksgiving service is being held shortly.*

We now have official printed news bulletins after years of whispered extracts and are awaiting Lord Louis' (Louis Mountbatten's) *arrival eagerly. The outlying working camps have concentrated round the Gaol area and we are packed like sardines. The hospital has over 2000 patients and there is a severe outbreak of gastroenteritis to complicate matters. We are pushing vitamin B etc into patients but there are several cases of sudden death due to heart failure which are baffling the experts.*

We follow all references to POWs in the news very carefully and there is much speculation as to our future as each successive speaker seems to have different ideas on the subject. It seems however that we will be taken back home as soon as possible by air or by sea as transport becomes available.

During this exciting waiting period we rush to the doorways every time we hear a plane in the sky hoping to see for the first time for over 3 years the tricolour that means liberation and freedom for us.

Chapter Ten

Epilogue

While Harry was waiting to be repatriated he wrote this letter home:

Sept 6/45

My dear Mam, Dad and all the family

How can I begin to express in this, my first letter home after 3½ years durance fairly vile, what has transpired during that time. So much has shaken the Silman frame that when we are gathered round the fireside in the old homestead and pass round the brandy, I will recount to you such tales that will make you rock on your heels, and you will begin to wonder whether or not you had given birth to a second Dumas or Munchausen.

I expect that so much will be written by so many by the time I get home, that it will only need my corroboration and a few personal details to set the seal. However, let me start with a few facts about me. I am exuding rude health and rice from every pore, and during the past four weeks have put on over 20lbs in weight. I spend most of my waking hours taking out the tucks in my pants. I am now back to my old weight and have regained my manly figure and vigour. One naturally loses weight on a restricted Asiatic diet such as we have been pushing back for the past four years, but there is now a superabundance of good food pouring in on us.

We have now had the ball and chain hacked off, and ships

and planes are daily unloading supplies and troops of all descriptions. We are slowly getting used to a non-POW life, and still feel embarrassed when a Nip salutes us. We are hoping to leave here in a few days and proceed direct to the UK, but things are very confused at the present and we do not know exactly what is to happen to us.

As you probably know, in spite of the strict censorship prevailing at the time, I was nabbed by the Nips in Feb 42, and have been resting here all the time except for a short trip up country to Thailand and Burma lasting 9 months, during which time we constructed a model railway.

This interim period of waiting before we are bunged home is being made very pleasant by all sorts of organisations doing their best to provide us with food, clothing, toilet requisites etc. and we look like being re-equipped from head to foot before we are through with these blokes.

I hope that all at home are in the pink, and although I have been away from no. 22 for nearly 4 years, expect to find it unchanged except for the books not being tidied and replaced in the bookcase, and Mam's teeth possibly in a different glass due to the other one being worn out. I imagine with the concentration of forces at no. 22, conditions may be a little crowded, but I wouldn't notice that now – interval for a spot of bitter laughter. I anticipate getting a few months leave (with pay) after my return to

England, before I recommence the daily toil. You might cut out the odd advert from the Wanted column – if anyone wants a doctor who has been sober and out of mischief for the past few years. I have done all sorts of jobs so am not very particular now.

Writing this letter has its difficulties as I am shooing away mosquitoes with one hand, stopping would-be purloiners of my ink bottle with the other and trying to concentrate in spite of 2 loudspeakers blaring out the news and events of the day. One of the things we appreciate most is listening to the BBC again, and getting a regular up-to-date news service. The Nips neglected to lay this on for us.

I will write again as soon as poss.

Love from Harry

Harry met his beloved wife Dorothea within a few weeks of his return to Leeds. She said that although he was jaundiced and very skinny, she fell immediately in love with him because he made her laugh. They were very happily married for nearly 60 years. His three children, Jackie, Marilyn and Alan, gave him the loving family life he had wondered would ever happen, and his contentment was later completed by cherished grandchildren and great-grandchildren.

He worked as a GP until he was in his mid 70s, and it is clear from the testimonials and letters he received on his retirement that he was a much-loved doctor.

Harry always played down the harrowing events of his wartime years with a dry sense of humour, as can be seen in his first letter home.

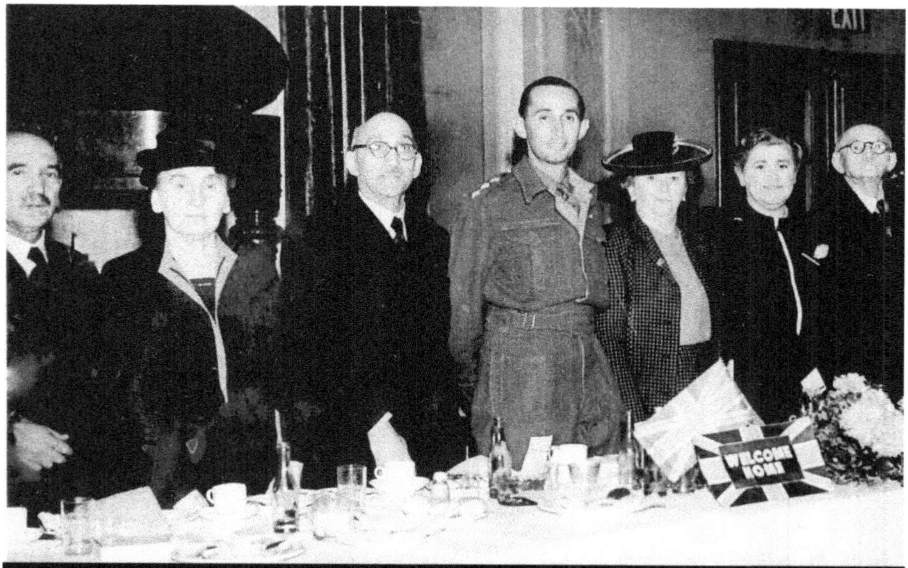

Welcome Home reception

I remember we were occasionally told we should finish what was on our plates as 'your father would have been very happy to have had a meal like this during the war', but otherwise our memories are of a cheerful person with a positive outlook on life.

When Harry died in 2005, he was not a fragile sick man of 94 but a kind, caring, funny human being who was an integral part of our lives. All the family would go to him for wise counsel, and until the very last few months of his life, he was always smiling, quick with a pun or corny joke. And, remarkably, still liked rice.

Appendix One

References

1. Yorkshire Television programme Back to the Front, a 2003 documentary chronicling the experience of six doctors in World War 2.

2. Louise Reynolds, daughter of Padre Eric Cordingly.
Down to Bedrock Ed (pub Art Angels 2013)
Echoes of Captivity Ed (pub High Winds 2020)

3. Paul Reynolds did comprehensive research on the RNF's time in France in the days leading up to the retreat from Dunkirk. His focus was his father-in-law, Padre Eric Cordingly attached, like Harry Silman, to the RNF for the whole of the war. Paul's research informed much of the content of my Chapter Two.

4. Padre Eric Cordingly
Down to Bedrock (pub Art Angels 2013)

5. Lieut Jim Bradley RE, fellow prisoner of Harry Silman.
Towards the Setting Sun (pub Phillimore 1982)

6. 'Fusilier George' author of A Story of the 9th Battalion, Royal Northumberland Fusiliers, April and May 1940. This is a personal and quite colourful account of the retreat to Dunkirk, probably written by one of the officers.

7. Official History of the Royal Northumberland Fusiliers 1952. I thank Paul Reynolds for giving me permission to use his research for the information from this History.

8. Montague Burton was a highly respected Leeds businessman. He declined the offer to be Lord Mayor of Leeds but was knighted for services to industrial relations. Founded biggest tailoring business, Burton Menswear, which made a quarter of British military uniforms in WW2.

9. Bill Frankland, one of four veterans interviewed in Radio 4 programme, The Reunion: Far East Prisoners of War presented by Sue MacGregor, recorded 26 April 2015

10. G P Adams
No Time for Geishas (pub Corgi 1974)

Appendix Two

Abbreviations & Army Terminology

AA	anti-aircraft
ACG	Assistant Chaplain General
ARP	air raid precaution
atap	roofing material made from palm tree leaves
barracks	large building(s) to house soldiers
batman	officer's personal assistant
billet	soldiers' living quarters
BEF	British Expeditionary Force
Boches	Germans (from French slang)
C-in-C	Commander-in-chief
CO	Commanding Officer
conscripted	ordered or forced to join the army (opposite of enlist)
dixies	huge cooking pots for mass catering
Div/Divn	Division
enlist	volunteer/sign up to go into the army
HQ	Headquarters
Hun	German
IJA	Imperial Japanese Army
K	khaki
KD	khaki drill
Latrines	army toilets – the quickest to make were the deep trench type. These consisted of digging a deep pit or trench, and partly covering it with wooden planks. They were not as hygienic as the Indian style latrines which are the squat style of toilet seen widely in Asia today.

Mess	military dining room
MI	Medical Inspection (MI Room was equivalent to a surgery)
MO	Medical Officer (ie doctor)
NCO	non-commissioned officer. NCOs usually reach officer level by working through promotions unlike others who come in to the army at officer level
Nips	Japanese (from Nippon, the Japanese language)
OC	Officer Commanding
OR	Other Ranks ie the ordinary soldiers who ranked below officers
Padre	army chaplain
POW	prisoner of war
RAOC	Royal Army Ordnance Corps
RAF	Royal Air Force
RAP	Regimental Aid Post (ie first aid station)
RASC	Royal Army Service Corps
RE	Royal Engineers (also known as Sappers)
RNF	Royal Northumberland Fusiliers
RP	rice polishings
S	Singapore
Topee	lightweight helmet-shape hat to protect from sun
Warrant officer	highest level of NCO

Lightning Source UK Ltd.
Milton Keynes UK
UKHW021322310720
367486UK00004B/79

9 781910 133200